RAPID-SEQUENCE REVIEW
OF ANESTHESIOLOGY

RAPID-SEQUENCE REVIEW
OF ANESTHESIOLOGY

WITH TIME-LIMITED PRESSURE

WON K. CHEE, M.D.

Clinical Assistant Professor of Anesthesiology
Mount Sinai School of Medicine
New York

BUTTERWORTH-HEINEMANN

BOSTON OXFORD JOHANNESBURG MELBOURNE NEW DELHI SINGAPORE

Every effort has been made to ensure that the drug dosage schedules within this text are accurate and conform to standards accepted at time of publication. However, as treatment recommendations vary in the light of continuing research and clinical experience, the reader is advised to verify drug dosage schedules herein with information found on product information sheets. This is especially true in cases of new or infrequently used drugs.

∞ Recognizing the importance of preserving what has been written, Butterworth-Heinemann prints its books on acid-free paper whenever possible.

Library of Congress Cataloguing-in-Publication Data

Chee, Won K.
    Rapid-sequence review of anesthesiology: with time-limited pressure / Won K. Chee.
        p.   cm.
    ISBN 0-7506-9933-7 (pbk. : alk. paper)
    1. Anesthesiology--Outlines, syllabi, etc.   I. Title.
    [DNLM: 1. Anesthesia--methods--outlines. 2. Anesthetics--outline.   WO 218.2 C515r 1997]
    RD82.4.C47   1997
    617.9'6'0202--dc21
    DNLM/DLC
    for Library of Congress   96-50977
                                                                     CIP

British Library cataloguing-in-Publication Data
A catalogue record for this book is available from the British Library.

The publisher offers special discounts on bulk orders of this book.

For information, please contact:
Manager of Special Sales
Butterworth-Heinemann
313 Washington Street
Newton, MA 02158-1626
Tel: 617-928-2500
Fax: 617-928-2620

For information on all medical publications available, contact our World Wide Web home page at:
http://www.bh.com/med

10 9 8 7 6 5 4 3 2 1

Printed in the United States of America

For Susan

Table of Contents

Preface

Rapid-Sequence Review of Anesthesiology: With Time-Limited Pressure is a concise yet comprehensive review book in clinical anesthesiology. It contains factual information in clinical anesthesiology and arranges it in a rational manner. It is concise, which is the very strength and popularity of any review book. Yet, it is comprehensive enough to cover all the topics for review. No other review book is available that contains such succinct and relevant information in such a highly concentrated and clarified form.

For those who face the challenge of board certification, a concise yet comprehensive review outline is a welcome proposition. The need for board certification in anesthesiology today has become absolute in terms of job security, career mobility, and academic recognition. Despite the critical importance, no definitive review text has been available. Board candidates have had no other choice but to rely on multiple conventional textbooks for their review. The process of review in this manner can be haphazard, inefficient, and discouraging. They will find this book particularly useful as the time pressure limits them from approaching a major textbook for review.

Rapid-Sequence Review of Anesthesiology: With Time-Limited Pressure is not designed to provide new information in depth. It is not written to explain the rationales or concepts behind the theories, as many textbooks do. Nevertheless, it will be able to satisfy those who seek to consolidate their knowledge into a distillated, practical form.

In addition, *Rapid-Sequence Review of Anesthesiology: With Time-Limited Pressure* is designed for those who seek quick conceptual orientation in clinical anesthesiology through a simplified presentation. It is designed for those who are completely overwhelmed by the amount of information presented in major textbooks. This review book provides a sense of orientation in clinical anesthesiology to be used before navigating through the plethora of available information in the field.

Although the text is prepared with diligence and sincerity, I urge readers to maintain enough skepticism to recognize any misleading information created by oversimplification as well as inaccuracy. I disclaim any liability caused by direct or indirect application of the information in this book.

Finally, I would like to express my gratitude to Ms. Susan F. Pioli, the Director of Medical Publishing at Butterworth-Heinemann, who provided invaluable enthusiasm and support for this project. I also feel deeply grateful for the service rendered by my colleagues and residents, who have assisted me in providing patient care while I was preparing this book.

WKC
New York
September, 1996

Acknowledgments

The author wishes to thank the following individuals for their helpful comments:

TAMESHWAR AMMAR, M.D.
Assistant Professor of Anesthesiology
Mount Sinai School of Medicine, New York

JAMES B. EISENKRAFT, M.D., M.R.C.P. (UK), F.F.A.R.C.S.
Professor of Anesthesiology;
Director of Anesthesia Research
Mount Sinai School of Medicine, New York

ELLEN KAVEE, M.D.
Clinical Assistant Professor of Anesthesiology and Pediatrics
Mount Sinai School of Medicine, New York

ANDREW LEIBOWITZ, M.D.
Assistant Professor of Anesthesiology and Surgery
Mount Sinai School of Medicine;
Associate Director of Surgical Intensive Care Unit
Mount Sinai Medical Center, New York

PRITHI P. SINGH, M.D.
Clinical Associate Professor of Anesthesiology
Mount Sinai School of Medicine;
Associate Director, Department of Anesthesiology
Elmhurst Hospital Center, Elmhurst, New York

Abbreviations

A-a	alveolar-arterial		D&T	delirium & tremens
AAA	abdominal aortic aneurysm		DA	dopamine
ABC	airway, breathing, circulation		DBP	diastolic blood pressure
ABG	arterial blood gas		DIC	disseminated intravascular coagulopathy
ACT	activated clotting time		DKA	diabetic ketoacidosis
ACV	assisted-controlled ventilation		DM	diabetes mellitus
ADH	antidiuretic hormone		DOE	dyspnea on exertion
AF	atrial fibrillation		DPAP	diastolic pulmonary arterial pressure
ALS	amyotrophic lateral sclerosis		DVT	deep vein thrombosis
AR	aortic regurgitation		ECG	electrocardiography
ARDS	adult respiratory distress syndrome		ECT	electroconvulsive therapy
ARF	acute renal failure		EDV	end-diastolic volume
ASA	aspirin		EEG	electroencephalography
AS	aortic stenosis		EF	ejection fraction
ASD	atrial septal defect		EMD	electromechanical dissociation
ATN	acute tubular necrosis		ENT	ear-nose-throat
AV	atrioventricular		ESV	end-systolic volume
BBB	blood brain barrier		ETT	endotracheal tube
BP	blood pressure		FDP	fibrinogen degradation product
BPD	bronchopulmonary dysplasia		FEV	forced expiratory volume
BSA	body surface area		FFP	fresh frozen plasma
BT	bleeding time		FR	French
BUN	blood urea nitrogen		FRC	functional residual capacity
BV	blood volume		FVC	forced vital capacity
C	cervical		GA	general anesthesia
CA	carcinoma		GABA	gamma aminobutyric acid
CABG	coronary artery bypass graft		GFR	glomerular filtration rate
CAD	coronary artery disease		GI	gastrointestinal
CBF	cerebral blood flow		GU	genitourinary
CC	closing capacity		H&P	history & physical exam
CHF	congestive heart failure		HA	headache
CI	cardiac index		Hb	hemoglobin
CMRO$_2$	cerebral oxygen metabolic rate		HbA	hemoglobin, normal adult
CMV	controlled mandatory ventilation		HBF	hepatic blood flow
CNS	central nervous system		HbS	hemoglobin, sickle
CO	cardiac output		HBV	hepatitis B virus
COPD	chronic obstructive pulmonary disease		Hct	hematocrit
CP	cerebral palsy		HCV	hepatitis C virus
CPAP	continuous positive airway pressure		Hg	mercury
CPB	cardiopulmonary bypass		HIV	human immunodeficiency virus
CPD	cephalopelvic disproportion		HPV	hypoxic pulmonary vasoconstriction
CPK	creatine phosphokinase		HR	heart rate
CPP	cerebral perfusion pressure		HTN	hypertension
CPR	cardiopulmonary resuscitation		IABP	intra-aortic balloon pump
CSF	cerebral spinal fluid		ICH	intracranial hemorrhage
CT	computed tomography		ICP	intracranial pressure
CV	cardiovascular		ICU	intensive care unit
CVA	cerebrovascular accident		ID	internal diameter
CVP	central venous pressure		IDDM	insulin-dependent diabetes mellitus
CXR	chest x-ray		IGP	intragastric pressure
DI	diabetes insipidus		IHSS	idiopathic hypertrophic aortic stenosis

IM	intramuscular	PG	prostaglandin
IM	intermittent mandatory ventilation	PIP	peak inspiratory pressure
IOP	intraocular pressure	PND	paroxysmal nocturnal dyspnea
ITP	idiopathic thrombocytopenia purpura	PO	by mouth
IV	intravenous	PRBC	packed red blood cell
J	joule	PSV	pressure support ventilation
JVD	jugular venous distension	PSVT	paroxysmal supraventricular tachycardia
K	thousand	PT	prothrombin time
L	liter, lumbar, left	PTT	partial thromboplastin time
LA	left atrium	PVC	premature ventricular contraction
LAE	left atrial enlargement	PVD	peripheral vascular disease
LBBB	left bundle branch block	PVR	pulmonary vascular resistance
LES	lower esophageal sphincter	R	right
LFT	liver function test	RA	rheumatoid arthritis, right atrium
LMA	laryngeal mask airway	RBBB	right bundle branch block
LOC	loss of consciousness	RBC	red blood cell
LR	lactated Ringer's	RDS	respiratory distress syndrome
LSB	left sternal border	RLL	right lower lobe
LV	left ventricle	RML	right middle lobe
LVEDP	left ventricular end-diastolic pressure	RR	respiration rate
LVEDV	left ventricular end-diastolic volume	RSD	reflex sympathetic dystrophy
LVH	left ventricular hypertrophy	RT	radiation therapy
MAC	minimum alveolar concentration	RV	right ventricle, residual volume
MAO	monoamine oxidase	RVH	right ventricular hypertrophy
MAP	mean arterial pressure	S	sacral
MBC	maximum breathing capacity	SA	sinoatrial
MH	malignant hyperthermia	SBP	systolic blood pressure
MI	myocardial ischemia/infarction	SC	subcutaneous
MPAP	mean pulmonary arterial pressure	SF_6	sulfur hexafluoride
MR	mitral regurgitation	SIADH	syndrome of inappropriate ADH
MS	mitral stenosis, multiple sclerosis	SL	sublingual
MSO_4	morphine sulfate	SLE	systemic lupus erythematosus
MV	minute ventilation	SPAP	systolic pulmonary arterial pressure
MVP	mitral valve prolapse	SR	sinus rhythm
NE	norepinephrine	SSEP	somatosensory evoked potentials
NG	nasogastric	SV	stroke volume
NIDDM	non-insulin dependent diabetes mellitus	SVC	superior vena cava
NMJ	neuromuscular junction	SVR	systemic vascular resistance
NO	nitric oxide	SVT	supraventricular tachycardia
N_2O	nitrous oxide	T	thoracic, temperature
NPO	nothing by mouth	T&C	type & crossmatch
NS	normal saline	TB	tuberculosis
NSR	normal sinus rhythm	TBG	thyroid-binding globulin
NTG	nitroglycerin	TBW	total body water
N/V	nausea/vomiting	TCA	tricyclic antidepressant
OR	operating room	TEE	transesophageal echocardiogram
PA	pulmonary artery	TEF	tracheoesophageal fistula
PABA	para-amino benzoic acid	TFT	thyroid function test
PAC	pulmonary artery catheter	TIA	transient ischemic attack
PAP	pulmonary arterial pressure	TLC	total lung capacity
PCWP	pulmonary capillary wedge pressure	TMJ	tympanomandibular joint
PDA	patent ductus arteriosus	TOF	tetralogy of Fallot; train of four
PE	pulmonary embolism	TPN	total parenteral nutrition
PEEP	positive end-expiratory pressure	TSH	thyroid stimulating hormone
PFT	pulmonary function test	TTP	thrombotic thrombocytopenic purpura

TURP	transurethral resection of prostate
TV	tidal volume
URI	upper respiratory tract infection
VA	ventriculoatrial
VC	vital capacity
VF	ventricular fibrillation
VMA	vanillymandelic acid
V/Q	ventilation-perfusion
VSD	ventricular septal defect
VSS	vital signs stable
VT	ventricular tachycardia
WPW	Wolf-Parkinson-White

1

ABC PROBLEMS

☞ *Check ABC.*

Airway (hypoxemia?)
☞ *Administer 100% O$_2$.*
Breathing (hypercarbia?)
☞ *Listen to the patient for bilateral breath sound.*
Circulation (hypotension? hypertension? arrhythmias?)
☞ *Check BP, ECG.*

OXYGENATION PROBLEMS

the ASA standard monitors for oxygenation: a pulse oximeter, an oxygen analyzer

HYPOXEMIA

☞ *Check ABC.*

Hypoxemia occurs in <u>blood</u>.
Hypoxia occurs in <u>tissue</u>.

RELATIONSHIP BETWEEN PaO$_2$ AND SaO$_2$

PaO$_2$ (mm Hg)	26	40	50	60	97
SaO$_2$ (%)	50	70	80	90	97

MANAGEMENT

Administer 100% O$_2$.
Check vital signs on the monitors.
Manually ventilate the patient:
    Check for resistance (lung compliance).
    Rule out mechanical failure (circuit disconnection vs. ETT obstruction).
Check for bilateral breath sound and chest excursion.

CAUSES

☞ *Possible causes of hypoxemia include anything that may prevent oxygen molecules from traveling from the pipeline source to the patient's fingertip where a pulse oximeter probe detects the oxygen saturation level.*
The oxygen molecules travel through the ventilator, the endotracheal tube, the lung (into the blood), the heart and down to the tissue in a mechanically ventilated patient.

VENTILATOR
Low FIO_2:
  empty oxygen tank, hypoxic gas mixture
Mechanical failure:
  circuit disconnection

ETT
Obstruction:
  mucous plugs, kinks, herniated cuff, biting
Wrong position:
  esophageal intubation, endobronchial intubation

LUNG
Shunt:
  aspiration, atelectasis, bronchospasm, pulmonary edema, pneumothorax
Dead space:
  pulmonary embolism, amniotic fluid embolism, fat embolism

BLOOD
Deficit:
  anemia, hypovolemia
Defect:
  cyanide toxicity, carbon monoxide poisoning, met-hemoglobinemia, sickle cell crisis

HEART
Low CO:
  MI, CHF, shock, arrhythmias, tamponade
R to L Shunt:
  Tetralogy of Fallot (TOF), Eisenmenger syndrome, pulmonic atresia

PULSE OXIMETER
Artifacts:
  motion, ambient light, electrocautery, hypothermia, methylene blue

VENTILATION PROBLEMS

the ASA standard monitors for ventilation:
a capnography, a precordial stethoscope, a disconnection alarm

HYPERCARBIA

☞ *Check the patient.*
☞ *Check the ventilator.*

CAUSES

INCREASED CO_2 **PRODUCTION**

Hypermetabolism:
light anesthesia, fever, shivering, sepsis
MH, hyperthyroidism

External sources:
CO_2 insufflation, TPN

DECREASED CO_2 **ELIMINATION**

CNS problems:
hypoventilation   (neurologic, pharmacologic, metabolic causes)

Lung problems:
V/Q mismatch   (dead space/shunt)

Neuromuscular problems:
chest wall defect   (restrictive lung diseases, high spinal blockade)

Ventilator problems:
rebreathing   (low fresh gas flow, defective CO_2 absorber or unidirectional valves)
hypoventilation   (inadequate ventilatory settings, disconnection)

CIRCULATION PROBLEMS

the ASA standard monitors for circulation: a BP cuff, ECG

HYPOTENSION
☞ *Check ABC.*

MANAGEMENT
Administer 100% O_2.
Treat **Preload** deficit:
    IV fluid, Trendelenburg position
Treat **Afterload** deficit:
    vasoconstictors
Treat **Contractility** deficit:
    inotropes, antiarrhythmics

CAUSES
☞ *Remember by preload, afterload, contractility:*
Since   SVR = (MAP − CVP)/CO,
then,   MAP = (SVR × CO) + CVP.
Therefore, low MAP = (low SVR × low CO) + low CVP
*or   hypotension = (low **afterload** × low **contractility**) + low **preload***

PRELOAD DEFICIT
Volume deficit:
    blood loss, third-spacing (most common)
Venous obstruction:
    tension pneumothorax, positive pressure ventilation, PEEP, embolus,
    surgical compression of blood vessels, cardiac tamponade

AFTERLOAD DEFICIT
Vasodilation:
    sepsis, anaphylaxis, transfusion reaction, drugs, sympathetic blockade (spinal blockade)

CONTRACTILITY DEFICIT
Myocardium:
    arrhythmias, MI, CHF, contusion, rupture
Metabolic/endocrine:
    hypoxemia, hypocalcemia, hypoglycemia, acidosis, alkalosis, hypothermia
    hypothyroidism, adrenal insufficiency
Drugs:
    beta blockers, anesthetic overdose

BRADYCARDIA
☞ *Check ABC.*

MANAGEMENT
100% O_2
Atropine
Isoproterenol
Pacemaker

CAUSES
HEAD:
    increased ICP
NECK:
    vagal reflex, spinal shock
LUNG:
    hypoxemia
HEART:
    MI, heart blocks

Metabolic:
    acidosis, allergic reaction, hypothermia
Endocrine:
    hypothyroidism, adrenal insufficiency
Pharmacologic:
    beta blockers, anesthetics, Dilantin, potassium, calcium, digoxin

TACHYCARDIA

☞ *Check ABC.*

☞ *Beta blockade in hypovolemia can precipitate complete cardiovascular collapse.*

CAUSES

SYMPATHETIC ACTIVATION

Pain:

light anesthesia, bladder distension

Pharmacologic:

sympathomimetics, anticholinergics, histamine releasers,
allergic reactions, drug withdrawal (beta blockers, alcohol)

Metabolic:

hypoxemia, **hypercarbia**, hypoglycemia

HYPOVOLEMIA

Absolute:

hemorrhage, third-spacing, anemia

Relative:

tension pneumothorax, cardiac tamponade

HYPERMETABOLISM

Metabolic:

fever, shivering, sepsis

Endocrine:

hyperthyroidism, pheochromocytoma, carcinoid, MH, neuroleptic MH

TEMPERATURE PROBLEMS

the ASA standard monitor for temperature: a temperature probe

HYPOTHERMIA

CAUSES
Radiation: 60% through "*light*"
Evaporation: 20% through "*water*"
Convection: 15% through "*wind*"
Conduction: 5% through "*earth*"

EFFECTS ON ORGAN SYSTEMS
CNS
depressed mental status/airway reflex
decreased CBF/ICP, $CMRO_2$, MAC
HEART
arrhythmias, LV dysfunction, increased SVR
increased O_2 consumption with shivering
LUNG
increased PVR; decreased HPV
LIVER
decreased hepatic clearance
KIDNEY
increased diuresis from blunted response to ADH
BLOOD
increased viscosity, coagulopathy
L-shift of $Hb-O_2$ dissociation curve
acidosis, hyperglycemia

HYPERTHERMIA
☞ *Beware of CNS injury.*

CAUSES
Iatrogenic:
overheating
Inflammatory:
infection, sepsis, atelectasis, PE, allergic reaction
Metabolic/endocrine:
hyperthyroidism, pheochromocytoma, MH, neuroleptic MH

MENTAL STATUS CHANGES

"confused, agitated, unresponsive..."

☞ *Do not sedate without evaluating the patient.*
☞ *Check ABC.*

MANAGEMENT
Administer 100% O_2.
Check ABG, electrolytes.

CAUSES
ABC problem:
hypoxemia, hypercarbia, hypotension

Sympathetic:
pain (e.g., bladder distension), anxiety (e.g., ICU psychosis)

Pharmacologic:
anesthetics, including ketamine, atropine, scopolamine, droperidol
local anesthetic toxicity, $MgSO_4$ toxicity
alcohol/alcohol withdrawal, steroid

Metabolic/endocrine:
hyponatremia, hypoglycemia/hyperglycemia, uremia
hypothermia, sepsis, porphyria
hypothyroidism/hyperthyroidism, adrenal insufficiency

Neurologic:
CVA, meningitis, seizures

CARDIOPULMONARY RESUSCITATION (CPR)

☞ *Continuous ECG monitoring and IV access should be established for all patients.*
☞ *Chest compression, epinephrine, and an ETT are indicated when no pulse is present.*
☞ *Defibrillation is indicated for a rapid ventricular rate with cerebral/cardiac hypoperfusion.*

SUMMARY OF ALGORITHMS

Rhythm	Shock	ETT	Epi-nephrine	Atropine	Lidocaine	Other Antiarrhythmics	Pacing	Comments
VF/VT no pulse	200 J, 300 J, 360 J	yes	1 mg q5min		1 mg/kg q8min × 3	bretylium 5, 10 mg/kg over 10 min		Repeat shock after each drug. NaHCO$_3$?
VT with pulse	If unstable, 100 J, 200 J, 360 J syn.				1 mg/kg q8min × 3	procainamide 20 mg/min (max. 1000mg) bretylium 5, 10 mg/kg		precordial thump in witnessed arrest NaHCO$_3$?
Asystole		yes	1 mg q5min	1 mg q5min			yes	NaHCO$_3$?
EMD		yes	1 mg q5min					Treat the cause.* NaHCO$_3$?
Bradycardia AV blocks				1 mg × 2		isoproterenol 2-10 µg/min	yes	digoxin toxicity?
PSVT	If unstable, 100 J, 200 J, 360 J syn.					adenosine verapamil** beta blockers	yes	vagal maneuvers

* hypoxemia, acidosis, hypovolemia, cardiac tamponade, tension pneumothorax, PE
**contraindicated for WPW syndrome

2

DIFFICULT AIRWAY

☞ *Avoid muscle relaxants if the ability to intubate & ventilate the patient is uncertain.* Risk for aspiration is increased.

RECOGNITION & ANTICIPATION

MALLAMPATI CLASSIFICATION (1985)*

Class	Visual Exam of Pharynx	Vocal Cord Visualization
1	**Tonsillar pillars** and the rest of the parts below	yes
2	**Uvula** and the rest of the parts below	yes
3	**Soft palate** and the rest of the part below	no
4	**Hard palate** only	no

*does not evaluate the chin or the neck.

PHYSICAL CHARACTERISTICS

Uvula:
    invisible
Tongue:
    large
Mouth:
    small opening (<3 finger breadths), TMJ disease
Teeth:
    protruding upper incisors
Chin:
    receding, short distance (<6.5 cm) between mandible to thyroid cartilage
Neck:
    short, bulky, C-spine instability

COEXISTING CONDITIONS ASSOCIATED WITH DIFFICULT AIRWAYS

ACQUIRED
obesity
pregnancy
face & neck injury (trauma/burn injury, tracheostomy, radiation therapy)
neck mass (goiter from thyroid diseases, tumor, hematoma, abscess)
acromegaly
rheumatoid arthritis
epiglottitis

CONGENITAL
Down syndrome
Goldenhar syndrome
Pierre Robin syndrome
Treacher Collins syndrome

MANAGEMENT

☞ *Avoid muscle relaxants if the ability to intubate & ventilate the patient is uncertain.*
☞ *Call for help!*

OPTIONS

☞ *"Awake-look" may help assessing the level of difficulty in visualizing the vocal cords.*
☞ *Consider regional anesthesia, but anticipate complications.*

NON-EMERGENCY
☞ *Wake up the patient if possible.*
awake fiberoptic intubation/Bullard laryngoscopy
blind nasal intubation (contraindicated if facial fracture or coagulopathy is present)
retrograde intubation

EMERGENCY
(unable to intubate & ventilate)
laryngeal mask airway/Combitube
cricothyrotomy/translaryngeal jet ventilation
tracheostomy

AIRWAY INNERVATIONS AND BLOCKS

Vagus innervates larynx below the epiglottis.

INNERVATIONS OF LARYNX

BRANCHES OF VAGUS	SENSORY	MOTOR	LANDMARKS
Superior laryngeal nerve	above the vocal cord (internal branch)	cricothyroid (external branch)	corni of hyoid thyroid cartilage
Recurrent laryngeal nerve	below the vocal cord	all laryngeal muscles except cricothyroid	cricoid thyroid cartilage

LARYNGEAL MASK AIRWAY (LMA)

does not protect the airway.
is contraindicated in "full-stomach" (obesity, hiatal hernia).
allows positive pressure ventilation with PIP <20 cm H_2O.

LMA	Cuff	Patient
1	5 ml	neonate (<6.5 kg)
2	10 ml	infant (<20 kg)
2.5	15 ml	toddler (<30 kg)
3	20 ml	child, small adult
4	30 ml	adult

Rapid-Sequence Review of Anesthesiology

3

MALIGNANT HYPERTHERMIA

PATHOPHYSIOLOGY
hypermetabolism of skeletal muscles from failed Ca^{++} reuptake to sarcoplasmic reticulum (prolonged excitation-contracture coupling)

TRIGGERING FACTORS
Drugs: succinylcholine, inhalational agents (except N_2O)
Stress: exercise, surgery

INCIDENCE
1:50,000 in adults
1:15,000 in children

RISK FACTORS
☞ *Past history of general anesthesia without the complication does not rule out the present risk.*

Family history:
    autosomal dominant on chromosome 19 with mixed penetrance
Masseter spasm (trismus) with succinylcholine:
    Eliminate triggering agents.
☞ *Whether to continue with the surgery is controversial.*
    Monitor [CPK] for 24 hours.
Muscular diseases:
    muscular dystrophy, myotonic dystrophy (?), osteogenesis imperfecta, strabismus

DIAGNOSIS
[CPK] >20,000 IU:
    unreliable
Muscle biopsy for halothane-caffeine contracture test:
    First-degree relatives of known a MH patient should be tested.
    There are false-negative test results.
☞ *The biopsy result probably would not change the anesthetic management; and, therefore, would be unnecessary.*

MANAGEMENT

☞ *Do not jump to a conclusion; rule out other causes of hyperthermia.*

SIGNS & SYMPTOMS*	TREATMENT
Tachycardia (earliest)	Shut off and eliminate the triggering agent.
Hypercarbia (most sensitive/specific)	Hyperventilate.
Hypoxia	100% O_2
Acidosis	$NaHCO_3$/Check ABG.
Hyperkalemia	Insulin/D50W
Arrhythmias	Lidocaine/procainamide
Hyperthermia (late sign)	Cold IV fluid/cooling lavage till 38°C
Muscle rigidity	Dantrolene** 2.5 mg/kg q5min × 4
Renal failure (myoglobinuria)	IV fluid, mannitol/furosemide for urine output >2 ml/kg/h
DIC	Check PT/PTT, [fibrinogen], [FDP] FFP, platelets
Multi-organ system failure and death	MORTALITY: <5% with early treatment

* Muscle rigidity, myoglobinuria and metabolic acidosis are more prominent in MH
   than in thyroid storm or sepsis.

**Dantrolene:
   decreases intracellular [Ca^{++}] release by sarcoplasmic reticulum.
   potentiates muscle relaxation.
   crosses placenta and causes uterine atony.
   Pretreatment is not recommended.

4

PREGNANCY

ANESTHETIC CONCERNS
MAC decreases:
☞ *Reduce the drug dosages.*
FRC decreases:
☞ **Preoxygenate** *well.*
Aortocaval hypotensive syndrome:
☞ *Remember **left uterine displacement** after the second trimester.*
Full stomach:
☞ *Pretreat with **Bicitra**.*
Fetus and nonobstetric surgery:
☞ *Avoid N_2O (?) and **benzodiazepines** during the first trimester.*

FETAL HEART RATE DECELERATIONS
☞ *Monitor the fetal heart rate after 16 weeks gestation.*
Normally 120-160/min with beat-to-beat variability of 5-20/min

TYPE	MECHANISM	SIGNIFICANCE
Early	vagal reflex to head compression	normal
Late	uteroplacental insufficiency	fetal distress
Variable	umbilical cord compression	possible fetal distress

PAIN PATHWAYS

Stage	Innervation	Nerve block	Complication
1	uterus & cervix by visceral afferent (T10-L1)	paracervical	fetal bradycardia
2	vagina & perineum by pudendal nerve (S2-S4)	pudendal	a high failure rate

PHYSIOLOGIC CHANGES

Most changes occur during the first trimester.

CNS

Anesthetic requirement decreases:

Progesterone and endorphin decrease MAC.

Engorged epidural veins and increased abdominal pressure spread the local anesthetics to a higher dermatomal level.

AIRWAY

Airway becomes edematous➡Intubation could be difficult.

☞ *Do not lose the mother's airway to save the fetus.*

LUNG

MV increases:

TV increases➡PCO_2 decreases; yet pH remains normal.

FRC decreases; O_2 consumption increases➡Patient desaturates rapidly.

HEART

CO increases:

The greatest increase occurs immediately after the delivery.

BV/SV increase➡Hct decreases by dilution.

SVR, MAP decrease.

CVP/PCWP remain unchanged.

GI

Risk for aspiration increases after the first trimester:

Gastric juice is more acidic and larger in volume.

LES tone is decreased; intragastric pressure is increased; gastric emptying is slower.

KIDNEY

GFR increases➡[BUN] and [creatinine] decrease.

$[HCO_3^-]$ decreases➡pH is still normal.

LIVER

[Pseudocholinesterase] decreases➡but not significant for succinylcholine metabolism.

[alkaline phosphatase] increases.

PREECLAMPSIA & ECLAMPSIA

Etiology is unclear:
> uteroplacental ischemia-induced release of renin/angiotensin
> an imbalance between thromboxane and prostacyclin

Triad for diagnosis:
> **hypertension** (>140/90 or >30/15 mm Hg increase from baseline BP)
> **proteinuria** (>500 mg/day)
> **edema** (hand, face)
> occurring after 20 weeks gestation

Risk factors:
> "young," first pregnancy, "poor"
> diabetics, multiple gestation, polyhydramnios

MANAGEMENT
The most common cause of death is intracranial hemorrhage.

SYSTEM	SIGNS & SYMPTOMS	TREATMENT**
CNS	seizures (cerebral edema) headache (intracranial hemorrhage) visual disturbance (retinal detachment)	[MgSO$_4$] at 4-6 mEq/L
HEART	HTN CHF exaggerated response to vasopressers	hydralazine trimethaphan, digoxin, NTG A-line, CVP/PAC monitoring no epi in locals for epidural
LUNG	ARDS pulmonary edema airway edema	100% O$_2$/ventilatory support furosemide, NTG ABG, PAC monitoring
KIDNEY	oliguria, proteinuria, renal failure (fibrin deposit to basement membrane)	Maintain & monitor the urine output/volume status with a Foley catheter/PAC.
LIVER	increased LFTs* subcapsular hepatic necrosis/rupture	Monitor LFTs, PT/PTT.
BLOOD	thrombocytopenia* hemolysis* DIC	[PLT] >100 K for regional anesthesia Transfuse PLT, FFP.

* **HELLP** syndrome refers to **H**emolysis, **EL**evated **L**FTs, **L**ow **P**latelet count.
**The ultimate treatment is delivery.

DRUGS IN OBSTETRICS

UTERINE RELAXANTS

Name	Action	Dose	Side effects
$MgSO_4$*	Decreases acetylcholine release/sensitivity at NMJ. Muscle relaxation Sedation/anticonvulsant	4-6 g loading 1-3 g/h infusion	5 mEq/L: therapeutic/muscle relax** 10 mEq/L: decreased deep tendon reflex 15 mEq/L: respiratory arrest 20 mEq/L: cardiac arrest
terbutaline ritodrine	Beta$_2$ agonists: inhibit uterine contraction		hypotension, tachycardia pulmonary edema hypokalemia, hyperglycemia

* $CaCl_2$ antagonizes the effects of $MgSO_4$.

**Reduce the dosages for muscle relaxants and sedatives.*

UTERINE CONTRACTORS

Name	Class	Dose	Side effects
oxytocin (Pitocin)	a pituitary hormone	10-20 units/L	hypotension, water intoxication
Methergine	an ergot alkaloid	0.2 mg IM	HTN, CVA
PG F$_{2a}$	a prostaglandin	intrauterine injection	HTN, bronchospasm

ANALGESICS

Name	Dose	Comments
meperidine (Demerol)	10-25 mg IV 25-75 mg IM	less fetal respiratory depression than MSO_4 *Anticipate fetal depression if given <4 h of delivery.*
ketamine	10 mg IV bolus	uterine vascular constriction *Anticipate fetal depression if given >1 mg/kg.*

OBSTETRIC COMPLICATIONS

Risk is increased in multiparity.
Massive hemorrhage is involved.
GA with ketamine is preferred.

PLACENTA PREVIA

Pathophysiology:
   implantation of the placenta at the lower uterine segment

Onset:
   may occur any time

Risk factors:
   previous previa, "old" age, previous cesarean section

Signs & symptoms:
   painless vaginal bleeding (arterial)

☞ *Vaginal exam should be performed only with **"double set-up."***

PLACENTA ABRUPTIO

Pathophysiology:
   premature separation of the placenta

Onset:
   occurs after 20 weeks gestation

Risk factors:
   HTN, tobacco, cocaine use, uterinc anomaly, "old" age

Signs & symptoms:
   painful vaginal bleeding (venous)➡Massive bleeding may be hidden

☞ *Postpartum hemorrhage and DIC can occur*

UTERINE RUPTURE

Pathophysiology:
  rupture of the uterus

Onset:
  often occurs during labor

Risk factors:
  polyhydramnios, CPD, oxytocin, rapid labor, previous uterine incision

Signs & symptoms:
  sudden disappearance of the fetal heart sound, severe pain, shoulder pain

UTERINE ATONY

Pathophysiology:
  inadequate uterine contraction causing massive postpartum hemorrhage

☞ *Hysterectomy may be necessary to control the bleeding.*

RETAINED PLACENTA
☞ *Manual exploration under GA may be required.*

BREECH

Pathophysiology:
  "buttock-first" position

Risk factors:
  prematurity, polyhydramnios, twins, placenta previa

Complications:
  prematurity, birth trauma, maternal hemorrhage, mortality

TWINS

Complications:
    prematurity, breech, maternal hemorrhage

AMNIOTIC FLUID EMBOLISM

Risk factors:
    multiparity, "tumultuous" labor

Signs & symptoms:
    CNS   (seizures, coma)
    Heart (hypotension, asystole, EMD)
    Lung   (sudden dyspnea, hemoptysis, hypoxemia, bronchospasm)
    Other (DIC, uterine atony)

Treatment is mainly to support ABC.
Mortality is high.

MOLAR PREGNANCY (HYDATIDIFORM MOLE)

Pathophysiology:
    from abnormal placental growth

Onset:
    occurs before 20 weeks gestation.

Complications:
    massive hemorrhage, preeclampsia, hyperthyroidism, pulmonary emboli

☞ *Check TFT.* *

Remember that [thyroid-binding globulin], [T_3], and [T_4] are normally elevated during pregnancy, while [TSH], [free T_3], and [free T_4] remain unchanged.

5
OBESITY

DEFINITIONS
Obesity:
> > 20% over ideal body weight

Morbid obesity:
> >100% over ideal body weight

Pickwickian syndrome:
> chronic hypoventilation, hypoxemia, somnolence
> pulmonary HTN, RVH, cor pulmonale

ANESTHETIC CONCERNS
Difficulty airway:
☞ *Consider **awake intubation**; extubate wide awake.*

Full stomach:
☞ *Pretreat with Bicitra, Reglan, H_2 blockers.*
☞ *Perform **rapid-sequence** induction with cricoid pressure.*

Decreased lung volume:
☞ *Check ABG/PFT.*
☞ ***Preoxygenate**.*
☞ *Support post-op ventilation with adequate analgesia.*

CV abnormalities:
☞ *Check ECG, CXR.*

PATHOPHYSIOLOGIC CHANGES

CNS
Hypoventilation:
blunted ventilatory response to PCO_2
central sleep apnea

AIRWAY
Difficult airway:
massive pharyngeal soft tissues
limited neck mobility
large breasts

LUNG
Restrictive lung disease:
Decreased FRC,VC causes atelectasis, V/Q mismatch, hypoxemia, pulmonary HTN.
Decreased chest wall compliance increases work of breathing.

HEART
HTN, LVH, CAD, cor pulmonale
Increased BV/SV/CO

GI
Increased risk for aspiration pneumonitis:
Gastric juice is more in volume, lower in pH, slower in emptying.
Increased incidence of hiatal hernia, gastroesophageal reflux.

ENDOCRINE
Increased incidence of NIDDM.

OTHER
Increased incidence of DVT/PE.
Decreased dose requirement for local anesthetics in regional anesthesia.
Increased metabolism of inhalational agents:
Increased $[F^-]$ can cause renal toxicity.
halothane hepatitis (?)

6

COMMON UNCOMMON DISEASES

MYASTHENIA GRAVIS & MYASTHENIC SYNDROME

Muscle weakness caused by autoimmune processes

Prone to **respiratory failure** and **aspiration**
Risks for Post-op Ventilatory Support in Myasthenia Gravis (Leventhal et al. 1980),
(duration >6 years, pyridostigmine >750 mg/day, VC <40 ml/kg, COPD)

Abnormal responses to muscle relaxants:
☞ *Avoid muscle relaxants if possible.*

	MYASTHENIA GRAVIS	MYASTHENIC SYNDROME
AUTO ANTIBODY against	acetylcholine receptor of muscle endplate	calcium channel causing reduced acetylcholine release
COMPLICATIONS	heart blocks, cardiomyopathy respiratory muscle weakness	proximal limb weakness
SEX PREVALENCE	female	male
REFLEX	normal	decreased
with EXERCISE	weakening muscle strength	improving muscle strength
to SUCCINYLCHOLINE	*resistant*	sensitive
to NON-DEPOLARIZERS	sensitive	sensitive
ASSOCIATED with	thymus disease, stress	small cell carcinoma of lung
TREATMENT	anticholinesterases, steroids, plasmapheresis	4-aminopyridine

MUSCULAR DYSTROPHY & MYOTONIC DYSTROPHY

Hereditary muscle diseases:
☞ *Avoid succinylcholine.*
☞ *Avoid MH triggering agents.*

Associated with cardiac and pulmonary dysfunctions

	MUSCULAR DYSTROPHY	**MYOTONIC DYSTROPHY**
MUSCLE	weakness, atrophy	persistent contracture unresponsive to relaxants or anesthesia
HEREDITY	X-linked recessive (male)	autosomal dominant with variable penetrance
AGE	childhood	20-40 years
CNS	mental retardation	mental retardation, cataract, central sleep apnea
HEART	cardiomyopathy, MVP, MR	cardiomyopathy, MVP, heart blocks
LUNG	weak respiratory muscles kyphosis	weak respiratory muscles sensitive to respiratory depressants
OTHER		multiendocrine deficiency, uterine atony
Succinylcholine	**MH hyperkalemia**	**MH** *(controversial)* **prolonged muscular contracture**
MANAGEMENT	Prevent respiratory failure and aspiration. Consider regional anesthesia.	Prevent respiratory failure and aspiration. Avoid shivering. Avoid etomidate, anticholinesterases. Infiltrate with local anesthetics.

RHEUMATOID ARTHRITIS (RA), ANKYLOSING SPONDYLITIS, & SYSTEMIC LUPUS ERYTHEMATOSUS (SLE)

Airway management can be very difficult:

☞ *Consider awake fiberoptic intubation.*

Pulmonary dysfunctions include restrictive lung disease:

☞ *Check ABG/PFT, CXR.*

Cardiac dysfunctions include AR, heart blocks, pericardial effusion:

☞ *Check ECG, Echo.*

	RHEUMATOID ARTHRITIS	ANKYLOSING SPONDYLITIS	SYSTEMIC LUPUS ERYTHEMATOSUS
SEX	female	male	female
JOINT	symmetric cervical (C1-2 instability) cricoarytenoid TMJ	asymmetric total vertebrae sacroiliac TMJ	symmetric extremities cricoarytenoid
LUNG	pulmonary fibrosis pleural effusion	pulmonary fibrosis	pulmonary fibrosis pleural effusion
HEART	AR, heart blocks pericardial effusion	AR, heart blocks CHF	HTN, CHF, heart blocks pericardial effusion
OTHER	Rheumatoid factor+ conjunctivitis, renal failure platelet defect? (e.g., ASA)	HLA-B27+ conjunctivitis	ANA+ CNS disturbance renal failure, hepatitis

PORPHYRIA

PATHOPHYSIOLOGY
Excessive production of heme precursors from the defective synthetic enzyme activity,
resulting in **neurotoxicity**:

CNS changes	(mental status changes, SIADH with electrolyte disturbances)
autonomic dysfunction	(CV instability, GI disturbance)
peripheral neuropathy	(respiratory muscle weakness)

PRECIPITATING FACTORS
Metabolic:
> hypoglycemia, dehydration, sepsis, pregnancy

Pharmacologic:
> barbiturates, etomidate, ketamine, benzodiazepines,
> enflurane,
> Dilantin, alcohol, steroid,
> hydralazine, methyldopa, phenoxybenzamine

TREATMENT
glucose, hematin, beta blockers
cardiopulmonary support

SICKLE CELL ANEMIA

PATHOPHYSIOLOGY
Sickling of RBCs upon deoxygenation due to the abnormal hemoglobin (HbS),
resulting in vaso-occlusive crisis and multi-organ system failure as well as hemolysis.

PRECIPITATING FACTORS
Decreased tissue O_2 delivery:

hypoxia	(hypoventilation, anemia)
acidosis	(infection)
venous stasis	(hypotension, dehydration, hypothermia, tourniquet)

Increased tissue O_2 consumption:

stress	(fever, shivering, infection, sepsis, trauma)

TREATMENT
O_2, IV fluid, warming
Preoperative HbA RBC transfusion to achieve HbS <40%; Hct <40% (*controversial*)

7

KIDNEY PROBLEMS

Kidneys maintain fluid, electrolytes, acid-base balance, and drug excretion.
Minimal urine output should be 0.5 ml/kg/h.
Creatinine clearance estimates renal reserve most reliably.

CHRONIC RENAL FAILURE

Implies only about 10% of kidney function remains.
Abnormal volume status, hyperkalemia, and coagulopathy are common.
Uremia causes multi-organ dysfunctions.

BLOOD PROBLEMS

Anemia:

from erythropoietin deficiency and uremic bone marrow suppression.
Increased CO and R-shift of Hb-O_2 dissociation curve to maintain O_2 delivery.

Bleeding:

platelet dysfunction from the defective von Willebrand's factor and uremia.
☞ *Consider coagulation profile before performing regional anesthesia.*

Hypovolemia/fluid overload:

depends on the timing of dialysis
prone to HTN, CHF

Infection:

sepsis from leukocyte dysfunction
hepatitis from hemodialysis

METABOLIC PROBLEMS

Hyperkalemia:
☞ *Check [K⁺] within 6-12 h pre-op.*
Succinylcholine raises [K⁺] by 0.5-1 mEq/L and should be avoided if >5.5 mEq/L.
Cardiac arrest can occur.
ECG changes include widening of QRS, tall T waves.
Treatment includes D50W with 10 units of Regular insulin IV, $CaCl_2$, $NaHCO_3$,
hyperventilation, Kayexalate, and dialysis.

Hyponatremia:
Fluid overload may cause HTN, LVH, CHF.

Hypocalcemia:
Hyperparathyroidism results in fragile bones.

Metabolic acidosis:
from decreased excretion of H⁺.
R-shift of $Hb-O_2$ dissociation curve occurs.
☞ *Consider mechanical ventilation to avoid respiratory acidosis.*

UREMIC PROBLEMS

Neuropathy:
encephalopathy	(mental status changes)
autonomic neuropathy	(orthostatic hypotension, gastroparesis, nausea/vomiting)
peripheral neuropathy	(lower extremity injuries)

Effusions:
pericardial effusion	(pericarditis, cardiac tamponade)
pleural effusion	(pulmonary edema)

OLIGURIA

Urine output <0.5 ml/kg/h or <400 ml/day

The most common cause is hypovolemia.

URINE STUDY

	PRERENAL	RENAL
Urine [Na$^+$]	<20 mEq/L	>40 mEq/L
Urine osmolality	>500 mOsm/L	<400 mOsm/L
U osm/P osm	>2	<1
Urine S. G.	>1.015	<1.015
BUN/creatinine	>20/1	<20/1
ETIOLOGY	decreased CO (hypovolemia, CHF)	Acute tubular necrosis (ischemia, drugs, myoglobin, contrast)

MANAGEMENT

Rule out **postrenal** causes:
> Flush the Foley catheter with NS.
> Consider bladder perforation.

Rule out **prerenal** causes:
> Check urine electrolytes/osmolarity.
> Perform fluid challenges.

Consider **renal** causes:
> Monitor CVP/PCWP.
> Administer dopamine.
> Administer diuretics.

TRANSURETHRAL RESECTION OF PROSTATE (TURP)

☞ *Check pre-op [Na⁺]; delay the surgery if <130 mEq/L.*

☞ *Keep the resection time under 1 hour.*

☞ *Spinal anesthesia allows monitoring for mental status change from hyponatremia.*

TURP SYNDROME

Refers to the complications caused by massive fluid absorption,
resulting in **hyponatremia** and **fluid overload**.

The irrigation solution is absorbed from the open venous sinuses at the rate of >20 ml/min.

The rate of fluid absorption depends on:

    surface area of the open venous sinuses
    pressure from the irrigation bag to the patient
    duration of the procedure

Complications	Signs & Symptoms	Pathophysiology	Management
Hyponatremia	$[Na^+]$ < 120 mEq/L: CNS changes/seizure from cerebral edema $[Na^+]$ < 100 mEq/L: VF/VT	Massive absorption of the irrigation fluid causes hypervolemic, dilutional hyponatremia.	Stop the surgery. Support ABC. Administer Lasix; 3% NS if $[Na^+]$ <120 slowly (2 mEq/h) to avoid pontomyolysis.
CHF Pulmonary edema	hypotension HTN/bradycardia **hypoxemia** wheezing	same as above	Stop the surgery. Support ABC. Administer Lasix. Consider PAC.
Glycine toxicity Ammonia toxicity	transient blindness nausea/vomiting coma	The absorbed glycine potentiates GABA action on retina.	Stop the surgery. Support ABC.
Bladder perforation	hypotension shoulder pain (referred pain from diaphragm irritation)	surgical instrumentation	Suprapubic cystostomy
Bleeding DIC	hypotension	thromboplastin release from prostate	Aminocaproic acid to inhibit plasmin
Septic shock Bacteremia	hypotension fever/chills	surgical instrumentation	Support ABC. Antibiotics

8

VALVULAR HEART DISEASES

☞ *Rule out **CHF**, **coagulopathy** from anticoagulants.*
☞ *Remember prophylactic **antibiotics**.*
☞ *Take a careful history and physical exam.*

NYHA CLASSIFICATION OF HEART FAILURE (1964)

CLASS*	SYMPTOMS
1	none
2	with ordinary activity
3	with minimal activity
4	at rest

*   Monitoring with a PA catheter is appropriate for class 3 or 4.

SUMMARY OF MANAGEMENT

	RHYTHM	HR	PRELOAD	AFTERLOAD	OTHERS
AS	SR critical	normal	full	tight	Cardiovert if not SR.
MS	SR AF slow	slow	normal	tight SVR relaxed PVR	Cardiovert if PSVT occurs. Avoid pulmonary edema.
MR	SR, AF	fast	full	relaxed	Increase contractility.
AR		fast	full	relaxed	Increase contractility.
MVP		slow	full	tight	Decrease contractility.
IHSS	SR critical	slow	full	tight	Decrease contractility. Cardiovert if not SR.

AORTIC STENOSIS (AS)

LV pressure overload.

Increased risk for CAD, MI, sudden death.

☞ *Maintain SR and avoid vasodilation.*

SIGNS & SYMPTOMS

History:

angina (from LVH)

dyspnea (from CHF)

syncope (from low CO)

Physical exam:

a systolic ejection murmur at the 2R intercostal space

LAB

Echo:

valve area <0.8 cm^2 for severe disease (normally 2.5-3.5 cm^2)

pressure gradient >50 mm Hg

PAC:

PCWP < LVEDP

ECG:

LVH, Q waves

CXR:

prominent, calcified aorta

MANAGEMENT

Rhythm:

Maintain SR.　　("Atrial kick" contributes 50% of the SV.)

☞ *Cardiovert promptly.*

HR:

Avoid tachycardia (to maintain diastolic filling).

Avoid bradycardia (to maintain CO).

Preload:

Maintain volume.

☞ *Avoid NTG.*

Afterload:

Avoid vasodilation (to maintain coronary perfusion).

☞ *Avoid spinal anesthesia.*

MITRAL STENOSIS (MS)

LA/pulmonary pressure overload.

Increased risk for CHF, pulmonary edema, and systemic embolism.

☞ *Avoid tachycardia or vasodilation.*

SIGNS & SYMPTOMS

History:

rheumatic heart disease

symptoms of CHF (DOE, PND, orthopnea)

Physical exam:

a rumbling diastolic murmur, opening snap

signs of CHF (JVD, S3, rales, ascites, hepatojugular reflux, pedal edema)

LAB

Echo:

valve area <1 cm^2 for severe disease (normally 4-6 cm^2)

pressure gradient >10 mm Hg

PAC:

pulmonary HTN (MPAP >25 mm Hg)

PCWP > LVEDP

ECG:

LAE, AF, RVH

CXR:

prominent LA

MANAGEMENT

Rhythm:

Maintain SR or AF (if chronic).

☞ *Cardiovert if PSVT occurs.*

HR:

Avoid tachycardia.

☞ *Consider digoxin, esmolol, cardiversion.*

Preload:

Maintain volume.

Avoid pulmonary edema from fluid overload/Trendelenburg position.

Afterload:

Avoid pulmonary HTN.

☞ *Avoid hypoxia, hypercarbia, acidosis, or N$_2$O.*

Avoid vasodilation.

☞ *Avoid spinal anesthesia.*

MITRAL REGURGITATION (MR)

LA/pulmonary volume overload.

Increased risk for CHF, pulmonary edema, endocarditis, systemic embolism, sudden death.

☞ *Maintain "fast, full, forward."*

SIGNS & SYMPTOMS

History:

rheumatic fever, infective endocarditis, MVP

MI, trauma (e.g., " steering wheel" injury)

Marfan syndrome, osteogenesis imperfecta, Ehler-Danlos syndrome, muscular dystrophy

symptoms of CHF (DOE, PND, orthopnea)

Physical exam:

a holosystolic murmur at the apex (LSB)

signs of CHF (JVD, S3, rales, ascites, hepatojugular reflux, pedal edema)

LAB

Echo:

regurgitant fraction >0.6

PAC:

a prominent *v* wave on the PCWP tracing

PCWP > LVEDP

ECG:

AF (chronic) or SR (acute)

LVH

MANAGEMENT

HR:

 fast (to decrease the diastolic filling time)

Preload:

 full

Afterload:

 relaxed (to decrease the regurgitant fraction)

Contractility:

 forward

AORTIC REGURGITATION (AR)

LV volume overload.

☞ *Maintain "fast, full, forward."*

SIGNS & SYMPTOMS

History:

    endocarditis (IV drug abuse, sepsis)

    dissecting aortic aneurysm (trauma, syphilis)

    rheumatoid arthritis, ankylosing spondylitis

Physical exam:

    a decrescendo diastolic murmur

    a wide pulse pressure (SBP– DBP >40 mm Hg)

LAB

Echo:

    regurgitant fraction >0.6

PAC:

    PCWP < LVEDP

ECG:

    LVH

CXR:

    CHF

MANAGEMENT

HR:

    fast

☞ Avoid excessive tachycardia as LVH already increases O_2 consumption.

Preload:

    full

Afterload:

    relaxed

Contractility:

    forward

MITRAL VALVE PROLAPSE (MVP)

Usually asymptomatic, but MR, arrhythmias, sudden death are possible.

☞ *Avoid tachycardia or vasodilation. (Avoid sympathetic activation.)*

SIGNS & SYMPTOMS

History:

female

chest pain, arrhythmias (PSVT), embolism, endocarditis

Marfan syndrome, myotonic dystrophy

Physical exam:

a mid-systolic click (a high pitch systolic murmur)

LAB

Echo:

systolic prolapse of the mitral valve leaflet into the LA

ECG:

inverted/biphasic T waves in the inferior leads

MANAGEMENT

Rhythm:
SR

HR:
slow

Preload:
full

Afterload:
tight

Contractility:
soft

IDIOPATHIC HYPERTROPHIC SUBAORTIC STENOSIS (IHSS)

LV outflow tract obstruction.

☞ *Avoid tachycardia or vasodilation. (Avoid sympathetic activation.)*

SIGNS & SYMPTOMS

History:
> family history
> HTN
> angina, dyspnea, syncope (same as in AS)
> sudden death

Physical exam:
> similar to AS

LAB

Echo:
> hypertrophic LV septum
> anterior leaflet motion of the mitral valve into the outflow tract

ECG:
> LVH, Q waves

CXR:
> CHF

MANAGEMENT

☞ *Prevent LV emptying.*

Rhythm:
> *SR*
> ☞ *Treat SVT with cardioversion to maintain SV.*

HR:
> *slow*
> ☞ *Consider beta blockers, pacing.*

Preload:
> *full*
> ☞ *Avoid NTG.*

Afterload:
> *tight*
> ☞ *Use phenylephrine; avoid verapamil, isoflurane, MSO_4.*

Contractility:
> *soft*
> ☞ *Use halothane, beta blockers; avoid digoxin, ketamine.*

9

TRAUMA & ASSOCIATED INJURIES

"MVA, fall, burn, diving/drowning, found unconscious..."

RESUSCITATION
☞ Check and support **ABC**.
☞ Assume **full stomach**.
☞ Rule out **C-spine injury:**
    Lateral neck x-ray may not detect 10% of the injury cases.
    A good range of motion without pain virtually rules out the injury.

ASSOCIATED INJURIES
☞ *Recognize/optimize the associated injuries before the induction of anesthesia.*

HEAD/NECK
    CNS:
        intracranial hemorrhage, spinal cord injury, alcohol intoxication, drugs
    Airway:
        face/neck injury, burn
CHEST
    Heart:
        cardiac contusion, cardiac tamponade, dissecting aortic aneurysm
    Lung:
        pneumothorax, hemothorax, aspiration, pulmonary contusion, fat embolism
ABDOMEN
    GI:
        liver/spleen rupture
    GU:
        kidney contusion
EXTREMITIES
Musculoskeletal:
        pelvis/long bone fractures with fat embolism or massive hemorrhage

SPINAL CORD INJURY

☞ *Check and support ABC.*
☞ *Avoid succinylcholine (Day 2 on).*

ACUTE PHASE
Refers to the first month of the injury.
Steroid given during the early phase may improve the neurological outcome.

RESPIRATORY FAILURE
Can occur from diaphragmatic paralysis (C3,4,5) or intercostal paralysis (above T7), resulting in **hypoventilation**, **hypoxemia**, and **aspiration**.
☞ *Awake fiberoptic intubation or rapid-sequence induction with cricoid pressure is recommended because of the reduced cough reflex and full stomach.*
Consider tracheostomy.

SPINAL SHOCK
Flaccid paralysis occurs during the acute phase and lasts for a month.
It is characterized by loss of sympathetic tone below the level of injury, resulting in **hypotension & bradycardia**.
From the loss of vascular tone, vasopressor reflex and cardiac acceleration nerves.
☞ *Fluid and inotropes should be administered with central line monitoring.*

AUTONOMIC DYSFUNCTION
Can cause **arrhythmias**, **paralytic ileus**, and **hypothermia**.

CHRONIC PHASE

AUTONOMIC HYPERREFLEXIA
Spastic paralysis occurs about a month after the spinal cord injury (**above T7**).

Pathophysiology:
> uncontrolled sympathetic responses to the triggering stimuli to the area below the injury
> due to the sympathetic motor reflex at the spinal level that is no longer mediated by
> the inhibitory input from the higher cortical level

Signs & Symptoms:
> **hypertension & bradycardia**
> (from vasoconstriction below & carotid sinus response above the injury)
> **CVA, seizures, arrhythmias**
> muscle spasm, visceral spasm, sweating, skin flushing

Triggering stimuli:
> stimuli of skin
> distension of bowel/bladder

Treatment:
> spinal, epidural, and general anesthesia
> nitroprusside, tirmethaphan, alpha blockers

HYPERKALEMIA
Can result in VF or cardiac arrest if **succinylcholine** is administered
during the period of Day 2* to 2 years of the injury.

*Muscle endplate receptors proliferate within 2 days.

HYPERCALCEMIA
From bone resorption.
Can result in **renal failure** and **bone fractures**.

BURNS

☞ *Check and support ABC.*
☞ *Avoid succinylcholine.*

Rule of 9's (Figure 1)
   Is useful in assessing severity and prognosis of a burn injury.

Major burn is defined as:
   second-degree burn >25% of the area burned
   third-degree burn >10% of the area burned
   smoke inhalation

Prognosis depends on:
   age
   % of the area burned
   smoke inhalation

RESPIRATORY FAILURE may occur from various reasons, including:
   upper **airway edema** and obstruction
☞ *Recognize and intubate before the airway becomes difficult.*
   carbon monoxide poisoning (normal PaO_2 & SaO_2 reading; increased [carboxyhemoglobin])
   chemical pneumonitis from smoke inhalation (ARDS can develop in 2 days.)
   (Tracheostomy increases overall mortality in patients with burn injuries.)

CARDIOVASCULAR DERANGEMENTS may occur from various reasons, including:
   hypovolemic shock as a result of **evaporation** over the burned area and
   of **extravasation** of plasma and protein through leaky capillary membrane
☞ *Replace fluid loss according to **Parkland Formula** (4 ml/kg × % burned for 24 hours).*
   hypertension from increased release of norepinephrine
   (Hyperdynamic phase follows in 2 days and lasts for 1 month.)
☞ *Treat HTN with alpha-blockers.*

RENAL FAILURE may occur from various reasons, including:
   hypovolemic **shock** and hypoperfusion of the kidneys
   increased load of hemoglobin and **myoglobin** from massive hemolysis and muscle necrosis
☞ *Maintain urine output with hydration and diuretics;*
   alkalinize urine with $NaHCO_3$.

GI DERANGEMENTS

ileus, cholecystitis, acute duodenal ulcer (**Curling's ulcer**)

☞ *Use NG suction and H₂ blockers.*

METABOLIC DERANGEMENTS

profound **hypothermia, sepsis, DIC**

resistance to nondepolarizing muscle relaxants

hypermetabolism (may occur by day 2)

☞ *Consider TPN.*

ELECTRICAL BURNS man cause additional problems, including:

arrhythmias, spinal cord **demyelination**, massive **muscle necrosis**, bone fractures

☞ *Monitor ECG, urine output, and [K⁺] carefully for 2 days.*

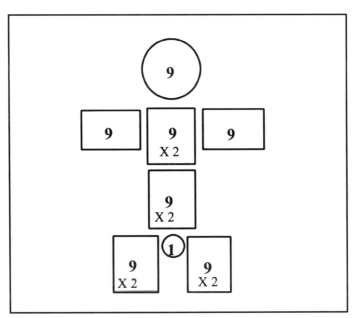

Figure 1. Rule of 9's

TRANSFUSION THERAPY

"When and why are you going to transfuse?"

To improve O_2 content
To improve coagulation

COAGULATION

COAGULATION FACTORS (12)
All are produced in liver except factor 8.

Fibrinogen (1)
Prothrombin (2)
Tissue thromboplastin (3)
Calcium (4)
Proaccelerin (5)
☞ *There is no Factor 6.*
Proconvertin (7)
Anti-hemophilic factor (8)
Christmas factor (9)
Stuart factor (10)
Plasma thromboplastin antecedent (11)
Hageman factor (12)
Fibrin-stabilizing factor (13)

COAGULATION INHIBITORS
Antithrombin 3 (needed for heparin to work)
Protein C
Protein S
Plasmin (degrades fibrin.)

COAGULATION PATHWAYS
Extrinsic: 3 (4)➡7 (4) ↘
Common: 10➡5 (4)➡2➡1 (4,13)➡FIBRIN CLOT
Intrinsic: 12➡11➡9 (8)↗

COAGULATION DISORDERS

HEMOPHILIA A
Pathophysiology:
    factor 8 deficiency
    X-linked recessive
Treatment:
    factor 8 concentrate, cryoprecipitate

HEMOPHILIA B
Pathophysiology:
    factor 9 deficiency
    X-linked recessive
Treatment:
    factor 9 concentrate, FFP

VON WILLEBRAND'S DISEASE
Pathophysiology:
    von Willebrand's factor deficiency
    autosomal dominant
Von Willebrand's factor:
    needed for platelet adhesion
    works with factor 8 as a complex
    produced in endothelial system
Treatment:
    DDAVP (an ADH analogue) promotes von Willebrand's factor release
    cryoprecipitate

IDIOPATHIC THROMBOCYTOPENIA PURPURA (ITP)
Pathophysiology:
    platelet destruction caused by antiplatelet antibodies
Treatment:
    platelet, steroids, splenectomy

THROMBOTIC THROMBOCYTOPENIA PURPURA (TTP)
Pathophysiology:
    platelet deficiency caused by abnormal platelet aggregation
Treatment:
    steroids, aspirin, exchange plasmapheresis, splenectomy

LAB TESTS

ABO , RH TYPING, & ANTIBODY SCREENING
Type specific:
  ABO & Rh typing (takes 5 minutes.)
  Risk for hemolytic reaction is 1:1,000.

Type & Crossmatch (T&C):
  ABO & Rh typing + all other antibody screening (takes 45 minutes.)
  Risk for hemolytic reaction is 1:10,000.

COAGULATION PATHWAYS
Extrinsic: 3 (4)➡7 (4) ↘
Common: 10➡5 (4)➡2➡1 (4,13)➡FIBRIN CLOT
Intrinsic: 12➡11➡9 (8)↗

Prothrombin time (PT):
  Checks **extrinsic** pathway (3➡7) + common pathway.
  Prolonged by **Coumadin**, which inhibits vitamin K-dependent factors (**2, 7, 9, 10**).

Partial thromboplastin time (PTT):
  Checks **intrinsic** pathway (12➡11➡9➡8) + common pathway.
  Prolonged by **heparin**, which activates antithrombin 3.
  Increases in hemophilia A (8), hemophilia B (9), and von Willebrand's disease.

Activated clotting time (ACT):
  Prolonged by heparin, which is reversed by protamine.

Fibrinogen level:
  <100 mg in DIC

PLATELET
Platelet count:
  < 20 K for spontaneous bleeding
  > 50 K for minor surgery (increased blood loss in surgery)
  >100 K for major surgery, regional anesthesia

Bleeding time (BT):
  Checks platelet function. (unreliable)
  Prolonged by Aspirin, uremia, and von Willebrand's disease. (normally BT <10 minutes)

COMPONENTS

PACKED RED BLOOD CELL (PRBC)
Volume:
> 250 ml/unit

Indications:
> to improve O_2 content

Each unit raises Hct by 3%.
Do not dilute in LR or D5W.
☞ *If two or more units of O negative type were given, do not switch back to the patient's ABO type.*

FRESH FROZEN PLASMA (FFP)
Volume:
> 250 ml/unit

Indications:
> DIC
> hemophilia B (9), antithrombin 3 deficiency

CRYOPRECIPITATE
Volume:
> 10 ml/unit

Indications:
> hemophilia A (8), von Willebrand's disease, and DIC

Contains factor 8 (100 units/unit of cryoprecipitate), von Willebrand's factor, and fibrinogen.

PLATELET
Volume:
> 50 ml/unit

Indications:
> platelet deficiency from dilutional thrombocytopenia, DIC, ITP
> platelet dysfunction from aspirin, uremia, von Willebrand's disease

Each unit raises platelet count by 5-10 K for a week.
Keep at room temperature.
Match the Rh status.

COMPLICATIONS

INFECTION RISKS
HCV: 1: 3,300 /unit
HBV: 1:200,000 /unit
H IV: 1:250,000 /unit

HEMOLYTIC TRANSFUSION REACTION
Risk: 1: 6,000 /unit
Mortality: 1:100,000 /unit
Etiology: clerical error in majority
complement activation

SIGNS & SYMPTOMS	MANAGEMENT
Hemolysis (HA, fever/chills, N/V, dyspnea) Hypotension, tachycardia	Stop transfusion; repeat T&C. Support ABC. Monitor [K$^+$] and ECG.
Acute renal failure (flank pain, hemoglobinuria)	IV fluid, mannitol/furosemide, NaHCO$_3$, dopamine
DIC	FFP, platelet

10

BABIES & CHILDREN

PHYSIOLOGIC FACTS

Pediatric anesthesia requires full understanding of the anatomic & physiologic differences.

DEFINITIONS
Prematurity:
> <38 week gestation or <2,500 g body weight

Neonate:
> up to 1 month old

Infant:
> up to 1 year old

AIRWAY
☞ *During intubation, rapid desaturation and bradycardia should be anticipated.*
☞ *Intubation may turn out to be difficult.*

AIRWAY ANATOMY
Head: large occiput (causes hyperflexion of the neck.)
Tongue: large
Neck: short
Larynx: anterior, cephalad (The cricoid cartilage is the narrowest point up to age 5.)
Epiglottis: stiff, long, slanted

ETT
☞ *Check for the gas leak at 15-25 cm H_2O.*
☞ *Use an uncuffed ETT for age <10 years old.*

Size :
> (4 + age/4) mm ID

Length:
> (12 + age/2) cm at the lip

ORGAN SYSTEMS
CNS
MAC is decreased in premies; increased in neonates/infants.

HEART
☞ *Treat bradycardia/hypotension with atropine.*
CO depends on HR as SV is fixed by the noncompliant LV.

LUNG
☞ *Anticipate rapid desaturation after induction.*
O_2 consumption rate is twice as high as that of an adult.
Alveoli are prone to collapse:
FRC/kg is not decreased compared with that of an adult, but
CC is closer to FRC.
Lung compliance is decreased, while chest wall compliance is increased.

KIDNEY
☞ *Administer D5 ¼NS IV.*
Kidney function is immature for the first 6 months of life.
Hypoglycemia/hyponatremia can occur in neonates.

OTHER
☞ *Keep warm.*
Hypothermia is more likely to occur from:
the increased surface area to body weight ratio
lack of shivering mechanism to generate heat
(instead, brown fat metabolism produces heat and norepinephrine)

Increased incidence of malignant hyperthermia compared with an adult.
Decreased incidence of halothane hepatitis compared with an adult.

APPROXIMATE PARAMETERS

AGE	HR±20	SBP	ETT	LARYN	HCT	GLUC	BV
Preterm	140	50mmHg	2.5-3.0	Miller 0	40-50%	>20mg/dL	100cc/kg
Neonate	120-140	60	3.0-3.5	Miller 1	55	>30	90
Infant	120	90	3.5-4.0	Miller 1	30+	>40	80

PRE-OP CONCERNS

PREMEDICATIONS

If the child is over 1 year old and uncooperative, consider...

DRUG	SEDATION	INDUCTION
midazolam	0.3 mg/kg intranasal 0.5 mg/kg PO	
ketamine	3-5 mg/kg IM (with atropine)	5-10 mg/kg IM (with atropine)
methohexital	10-25 mg/kg per rectum*	25-30 mg/kg per rectum 10 mg/kg IM

*Insert an 8 FR catheter 3 cm deep for rectal administration.

NPO RECOMMENDATIONS

AGE	CLEAR LIQUID	SOLID FOOD
under 6 months	2 hours	4 hours
6 month to 3 years	2 hours	6 hours
over 3 years	2 hours	8 hours

UPPER RESPIRATORY TRACT INFECTION (URI)

Delay the elective surgical procedure if <u>acute</u> or <u>systemic</u> signs are present:

T >101°F

abnormal findings upon auscultation

productive cough

purulent nasal discharge

PREMATURITY & ASSOCIATED PROBLEMS

APNEA SPELL

Signs & symptoms:
apnea >20 sec, bradycardia, cyanosis

Risk factors:
postconceptual age <**60 weeks**
Hct <30%
GA

☞ *Delay the surgery.*
☞ *Post-op monitoring for 12-24 h is required.*

INTRACRANIAL HEMORRHAGE (ICH)

Pathophysiology:
from immature autoregulation of CBF

Risk factors:
hypoxia, hypercarbia
hyperosmolarity (e.g., $NaHCO_3$)

RETROLENTAL FIBROPLASIA

Pathophysiology:
from irregular hyperplasia of retinal blood vessels

Risk factors:
post-conceptual age <**44 weeks**
body weight <1,500 g
PaO_2 >60-80 mm Hg

Preductal A-line:
Reflects PaO_2 at retina & brain.
Measures at R radial or temporal artery.
PaO_2 gradient >20 mm Hg from postductal PaO_2 implies persistent fetal circulation.

☞ *Maintain SaO_2 at the pre-op RA level (SaO_2 92-96%).*
☞ *In respiratory distress, administer 100% O_2 (brain before eye).*

Rapid-Sequence Review of Anesthesiology

PERSISTENT FETAL CIRCULATION
☞ *IV tubing should be free of air bubbles to avoid systemic embolism.*

Coexisting high PVR results in R to L shunt through the communications.
Decrease PVR:
Avoid hypoxemia, hypercarbia, acidosis.
Administer tolazoline, PG E_2, prostacyclin, isoproterenol.

DUCTUS ARTERIOSUS
Closes functionally by 1 day; anatomically by 1 month.
Patent ductus arteriosus causes L to R shunt in the presence of normal PVR.
Indomethacin closes the ductus.

FORAMEN OVALE
Closes functionally by 1 year; probe-patent up to 25% in adults.
Patent foramen ovale causes L to R shunt in the presence of normal PVR.

RESPIRATORY DISTRESS SYNDROME (RDS)

Pathophysiology:
from lack of surfactant

Signs & symptoms:
decreased compliance, alveolar collapse, R to L shunt, hypoxemia, pneumothorax

Risk factors:
<34 week gestation
Lecithin/Sphingomyelin <2/1

BRONCHOPULMONARY DYSPLASIA (BPD)

Signs & symptoms:
hyperactive airway, infection, decreased compliance

Risk factors:
previous respiratory complications with medical interventions

NEONATAL RESUSCITATION

APGAR SCORE
Is checked at first minute and fifth minute after birth.
Evaluates for asphyxia; predicts survival and neurological outcome.
Score ranges from 0-2 for each category.

Appearance:	*pink?*
Pulse:	*>100/min?*
Grimace:	*gag reflex, crying?*
Activity:	*good muscle tone?*
Respiration:	*spontaneous, crying?*

☞ *Score 0 - 3:* *Intubate!*
Score 8-10: Healthy !

APPROXIMATE PARAMETERS

AGE	HR±20	SBP	ETT	LARYN	HCT	GLUC	BV
Preterm	140	50mmHg	2.5-3.0	Miller 0	40-50%	>20mg/dL	100cc/kg
Neonate	120-140	60	3.0-3.5	Miller 1	55	>30	90
Infant	120	90	3.5-4.0	Miller 1	30+	>40	80

INTRAOSSEOUS ACCESS
Indication:
   emergency & age < 6 years old

Needle:
   18 G spinal needle with a stylet

Site:
   proximal tibia below the growth plate
   distal femur

Complications:
   growth plate injury
   infection

ABC

AIRWAY	Suction the nose, the mouth (and the trachea if meconium is present).
BREATHING	Stimulate for spontaneous breathing. If **HR<100, mask-ventilate** with 100% O_2. (RR40-60; PIP15-20cm H_2O) If **HR <80** after 30 sec, **intubate.**
CIRCULATION	If **HR <60**, start **chest compression** (120/min, 0.5" depression). If HR <80 after 30 sec, support hemodynamics pharmacologically.

MEDICATIONS

DRUG	DOSAGE	TOTAL DOSE*	COMMENTS
Epinephrine	10 µg/kg IV/IM 100 µg/kg ETT	0.3 ml	Use 1:10,000 solution for IV/IM. Use 1: 1,000 solution for ETT.
Naloxone	10 µg/kg IV/IM/SC/ETT	0.1 ml (0.4 mg/ml)	Consider if narcotic is given <4 h of birth. Beware of precipitating withdrawal symptoms if the mother is an addict.

NaHCO₃	2 mEq/kg IV
	slowly
		10 ml
		(4.2%)
			Beware of causing ICH.
			Normal fetal pH:
			    7.30-7.35 (umbilical vein)
			    7.25-7.30 (scalp)

D10W	3 ml/kg IV slowly	10 ml	Consider if [glucose] <30 mg/dL. Consider when the mother is a diabetic or the neonate manifests seizures.
IV fluid PRBC	10 ml/kg IV slowly	30 ml	Consider with cord compression, placenta previa, placenta abruptio.
CaCl₂	10 mg/kg IV slowly	0.3 ml (10%)	Antagonizes the effects of Mg^{++}. Monitor ECG.
Atropine	10 µg/kg IV/IM	0.3 ml (0.4 mg/ml)	Minimum dose is 100 µg.
Dopamine	10 µg/kg/min IV		
Isoproterenol	1 µg/kg/min IV		
Defibrillation	2 J/kg	6 J	Monitor ECG.

*approximate dosages assuming the neonate's body weight to be 3 kg

SPECIAL PROBLEMS

☞ *In general,*
*All the special problems require **awake intubation** and **post-op ventilatory support**.*
*The **pulmonary** problems require **spontaneous ventilation** for induction.*
*The **abdominal** problems require **NG suction**, pre-op **hydration**, and **no N₂O**.*

OMPHALOCELE & GASTROSCHISIS

Herniation of abdominal viscera outside the abdominal wall
results in severe dehydration, infection, hypothermia, acidosis, hypoglycemia.

	OMPHALOCELE	**GASTROSCHISIS**
SITE OF DEFECT	base of umbilical cord (midline)	anterior abdominal wall (lateral to midline)
HERNIA SAC	present	absent
CONGENITAL DEFECTS	common (75%) VSD, Trisomy 21, GU defect	uncommon
ETIOLOGY	autosomal dominant	intrauterine vascular accident
ASSOCIATED WITH	macroglossia	prematurity

MANAGEMENT
PRE-OP
    Optimize the medical problems: dehydration, infection, hypothermia, acidosis, hypoglycemia.
    Rule out other congenital defects.
    Establish adequate IV access as well as A-line, CVP monitoring.

INTRA-OP
    Keep the patient warm.
    Decompress the stomach with NG suction.
    Preoxygenate well.
    Intubate awake, or perform rapid-sequence induction with cricoid pressure.
    Avoid N₂O.
    Maintain hydration; monitor urine output.
    Monitor [glucose] for hypoglycemia; administer D10W.
☞ *After closing the abdomen, If CVP increases by >4 mm Hg,*
    or if the intragastric pressure (measured by a fluid-filled 12 FR tube) is >20 mm Hg,
    reopen the abdomen to facilitate ventilation and venous return.

POST-OP
    Maintain ventilatory support.
    Monitor [glucose] to avoid hypoglycemia.

EPIGLOTTITIS & CROUP

☞ *Epiglottitis can result in complete airway obstruction and death.*

	EPIGLOTTITIS	**CROUP**
AGE	3 to 6 years	3 months to 3 years
ONSET	abrupt (hours)	gradual (days)
SIGNS & SYMPTOMS*	dysphagia, dyspnea sniffing position, drooling anxious, toxic	hoarseness, barking cough nontoxic
NECK X-RAY	enlarged epiglottis (thumb sign)	subglottic narrowing (steeple sign)
PATHOGEN	bacterial (H. Influenzae B)	viral (parainfluenza)
INTUBATION	yes	probably no

*Both involve fever and inspiratory stridor.

MANAGEMENT OF EPIGLOTTITIS

PRE-OP

☞ *Do not disturb the patient; complete airway obstruction may occur at anytime.*
Transport to OR in sitting position with ENT standby for emergency tracheostomy.

INTRA-OP

Equipment and staff for emergency airway procedures should be ready before induction.
Perform inhalational induction in sitting position.
Maintain spontaneous respiration.
Start an IV, and administer atropine to reduce secretion and bradyarrhythmia.
Attempt direct laryngoscopy when the anesthesia plane is sufficiently deepened.
Use a smaller ETT for intubation.
Perform rigid bronchoscopy or tracheostomy if the airway is lost.

POST-OP

Maintain intubation until edema subsides (few days).
Continue antibiotics and racemic epinephrine/steroid therapy.

FOREIGN BODY ASPIRATION

Age:
  6 months to 6 years

Site:
  R main stem bronchus (most common)

COMPLICATIONS
Edible:
  fragmentation, chemical inflammation

Inedible:
  trauma, bleeding

SIGNS & SYMPTOMS
Obstruction:
  respiratory distress with/without CXR findings

Inflammation:
  fever, wheezing

MANAGEMENT
PRE-OP
  Check CXR.
  Delay the surgery till NPO >8 h if stable. (*controversial*)
  Premedicate with atropine to reduce secretion.

INTRA-OP
  Perform inhalational induction if spontaneous respiration is desirable.
  Consider rapid-sequence induction with cricoid pressure if full stomach.
  After induction, suction the stomach.
  Consider topical lidocaine (3 mg/kg).
  Be vigilant for hypoxia, hypercarbia, arrhythmias, pneumothorax.
☞ *If total obstruction occurs at trachea by the foreign body,*
  push it back into the main bronchus.

POST-OP
  Be vigilant for airway edema and obstruction.
  Apply humidified O_2, racemic epinephrine, and dexamethasone (0.5 mg/kg).

CONGENITAL DIAPHRAGMATIC HERNIA

☞ *Pneumothorax, pneumothorax, pneumothorax...*

Pulmonary hypoplasia, pulmonary HTN, LV hypoplasia are involved.
Other congenital problems include polyhydramnios, spina bifida, ASD, VSD, TEF.

SIGNS & SYMPTOMS
Hypoxia:
   cyanosis, respiratory distress

Chest:
   barrel-shaped
   diminished breath sound, displaced heart sound
   bowel sound present

Abdomen:
   scaphoidal
   diaphragmatic respiration
   bowel sound absent

MANAGEMENT
PRE-OP
☞ *Do not mask-ventilate to avoid pneumothorax and further distension of the stomach.*
   Intubate awake; maintain PIP at 25-30 cm H_2O.
   Decompress stomach via NG suction.
   Establish a preductal A-line, CVP, additional IVs.

INTRA-OP
   Treat pulmonary HTN:
      Avoid N_2O, hypoxia, hypercarbia, acidosis.
      Consider pulmonary vasodilators (NTG, tolazoline, isoproterenol, PG E_1).
   Administer 100% O_2, fentanyl 20 μg/kg, a nondepolarizing muscle relaxant.
   Be vigilant for tension pneumothorax:
      Sudden hypotension, hypoxia with increased PIP.
      Consider prophylactic bilateral chest tube insertion.
   ☞ *Do not attempt to expand the contralateral lung.*

POST-OP
   Maintain ventilatory & circulatory support.
   Consider extracorporeal membrane oxygenation (ECMO)
   if not responsive to pharmacologic support.

NECROTIZING ENTEROCOLITIS
☞ *volume, volume, volume...*

Onset:
> first week of age

Risk factors:
> prematurity (<32 weeks), low birth weight (<1,500 g),
> asphyxia, infection,
> umbilical artery catheterization, exchange transfusion, hyperosmolar feeding

SIGNS & SYMPTOMS
Bowel ischemia:
> abdominal distension, bloody stools, pneumatosis intestinalis on x-ray

Metabolic problems:
> metabolic acidosis, shock, hyperkalemia, DIC

MANAGEMENT
PRE-OP
☞ *Establish adequate IV access; optimize volume status.*
> Establish an A-line; assess acid-base status, pulmonary status (RDS?), coagulopathy.
> Obtain blood components for transfusion.

INTRA-OP
> Intubate awake or perform rapid-sequence induction with cricoid pressure,
> using ketamine or fentanyl and a nondepolarizing muscle relaxant.
> Avoid N_2O.
> Maintain adequate hydration.
> (Over 100 ml/kg may be required to maintain the urine output of >1 ml/kg/h.)
> Prevent hypothermia.
> Maintain Hct >40%.

POST-OP
> Maintain volume resuscitation, ventilatory support.
> Administer antibiotics, TPN.

TRACHEOESOPHAGEAL FISTULA (TEF)

VATER syndrome:
    Vertebral defects/VSD
    Anal atresia
    TEF
    Esophageal atresia
    Radial/Renal anomalies

Metabolic derangements:
    aspiration, dehydration, acidosis, hypoglycemia

Congenital defects:
    CV, GI, GU

Risk factors:
    polyhydramnios, prematurity

SIGNS & SYMPTOMS
Respiratory distress with feeding:
    cyanosis, choking, coughing

Obstruction :
    excessive salivation, inability to pass a catheter orally

MANAGEMENT
PRE-OP
    Rule out other congenital defects; check ECG, echocardiogram, CXR.
    Treat aspiration, dehydration, acidosis, hypoglycemia.
    Establish IV access, a preductal A-line, especially for thoracic approach.
    Consider gastrostomy to decompress the stomach.

INTRA-OP
    Intubate awake; maintain spontaneous ventilation.
☞ *Position the ETT between the fistula and the carina by withdrawing*
    from the R main stem bronchus while listening to the breath sound at the stomach.
    Be vigilant for airway compression, lung compression, and heart compression by surgeon.

POST-OP
    Be vigilant for tracheal collapse after extubation, air leak at the anastomosis, pneumothorax.

PYLORIC STENOSIS

a medical emergency, not a surgical emergency
dehydration, pH/electrolyte derangements, **full stomach**

Pathophysiology:
hypertrophy of pylorus muscle fibers with submucosal edema

Onset:
usually 1 month old

Risk factor:
male, parent with the history

SIGNS & SYMPTOMS

Obstruction:
projectile vomiting

Metabolic derangements:
hypokalemic, hypochloremic metabolic alkalosis

MANAGEMENT

PRE-OP

Treat metabolic derangements:
IV hydration, electrolyte replacement.

☞ *Delay the surgery until medically optimized:*
VSS
pH 7.30-7.50
$[K^+] >3.0$ mEq/L, $[Cl^-] >90$ mEq/L, $[NaHCO_3^-] <30$ mEq/L
urine output >1 ml/kg/h

INTRA-OP

Decompress the stomach with NG suction.
Intubate awake or perform rapid-sequence induction with cricoid pressure.
Avoid hypocarbia, which exacerbates metabolic alkalosis and hypokalemia.

POST-OP

Be vigilant for respiratory depression from reactive hypoventilation to alkalosis.
Administer glucose IV to avoid hypoglycemia until good PO intake.

11

LIVER PROBLEMS

Acute hepatitis is associated with high post-op mortality.
The goal is to maintain hepatic blood flow.
The closer to the liver the surgical procedure is, the higher the post-op complication rate.

PHYSIOLOGIC FACTS

LIVER FUNCTIONS
SYNTHESIS
Glucose:
☞ *Monitor [glucose] to avoid hypoglycemia.*
Clotting factors (except factor 8):
☞ *Check PT/PTT.*
Albumin:
<3.5 g/dL worsens ascites;
<2.5 g/dL increases active drug portion.

METABOLISM
Drugs/toxins:
☞ *Reduce anesthetic dosages.*
Bilirubin:
Jaundice (>3 mg/dL) may be prehepatic, hepatic or posthepatic.

HEPATIC BLOOD FLOW
Hepatic blood flow is decreased by hypoxia, hypocarbia, hypotension, surgery, anesthesia.

Hepatic artery:
Supplies 30% of blood and 50% of O_2.
Directly proportional to MAP.

Portal vein:
Supplies 70% of blood and 50% of O_2.
Inversely proportional to splanchnic vascular resistance.

HALOTHANE HEPATITIS

Incidence:
1: 35,000 in adults
1:100,000 in children

Risk factors:
"Forty, Fat, Female," repeated exposures to halothane within *"Four weeks"*

Pathophysiology:
an autoimmune response
(formation of an antibody against a halothane metabolite-liver antigen complex)

JAUNDICE (> 3 mg/dL)

	ETIOLOGY	LFTS ELEVATED
PREHEPATIC	Hemolysis (hematoma, transfusion)	Indirect Bili (unconjugated)
HEPATIC	Hepatocellular injury from: drug (including alcohol, halothane) virus (HBV, HCV) hypoxia (CHF, shock, sepsis)	Indirect Bili (unconjugated) Direct Bili (conjugated) SGOT (AST), SGPT (ALT)
POSTHEPATIC	Biliary obstruction (stones, pancreatitis)	Direct Bili (conjugated) Alkaline Phosphatase

CHILD'S CLASSIFICATION (1964)

PHYSICAL SIGNS/LABS	GROUP A	GROUP B	GROUP C
ENCEPHALOPATHY	0	+	++
ASCITES	0	+	++
NUTRITIONAL STATUS	excellent	good	poor
[ALBUMIN] (g/dL)	>3.5	3.0-3.5	<3.0
PT PROLONGED (sec)	<3	3-6	>6
[TOTAL BILIRUBIN] (mg/dL)	<2	2-3	>3
MORTALITY	<5%	25%	>50%

CIRRHOSIS

Results in portal hypertension, ascites, coagulopathy, hypoglycemia.
Consider paracentesis for massive ascites.
LFTs may be normal.

CAUSES
Pharmacologic:
   alcohol
Infectious:
   chronic active hepatitis
Metabolic:
   primary biliary cirrhosis, hemochromatosis, Wilson's disease

PATHOPHYSIOLOGIC CHANGES

CNS
depressed mental status/airway reflex
encephalopathy from NH_4^+ buildup, alcohol
hypoglycemia from impaired glucose synthesis
decreased **albumin** level to bind active drugs; decreased drug metabolism

HEART
hyperdynamic circulation (increased CO, decreased SVR) from anemia
arrhythmias
cardiomyopathy and CHF from alcohol and sodium & water retention

LUNG
hypoxemia
restrictive disease from **ascites**
R to L intrapulmonary **shunt** from portal HTN

GI
full stomach from autonomic neuropathy
duodenal ulcer, gallstones from biliary stasis
esophageal varices from portal HTN

KIDNEY
prone to failure (**hepatorenal syndrome**)
increased V_d from resorption of Na^+/ H_2O

BLOOD
coagulopathy from decreased production of clotting factors, splenic platelet sequestration
sepsis from infection, decreased immunity from leukocytopenia
hypothermia from decreased nonshivering thermogenesis

12

ENDOCRINE PROBLEMS

DIABETES MELLITUS (DM)

☞ *Evaluate other organ system dysfunctions.*
☞ *Rule out ketoacidosis.*
☞ *Maintain [glucose] at 100-200 mg/dL.*

IDDM vs. NIDDM

	IDDM (Type I)	NIDDM (Type II)
ONSET	"juvenile"	after 30s
RISK FACTOR	genetic	obesity
PATHOPHYSIOLOGY	lack of insulin	insensitivity to insulin
COMPLICATIONS	**micro**vascular sclerosis ketoacidosis	**macro**vascular sclerosis hyperosmolar nonketotic coma
TREATMENT	insulin	oral hypoglycemic agents

INSULINS/ ORAL HYPOGLYCEMIC AGENTS

Insulins do not cross placenta; oral hypoglycemic agents cross placenta.

AGENT	DURATION	ONSET/PEAK
Regular insulin	6 h	0.5 h/2 h
NPH, Lente	1 day	2 h/6 h
Micronase (glyburide)	1 day	1 h
Glucotrol (glipizide)	1 day	1 h
Diabinese (chlorpropamide)	3 days	2 h

ORGAN SYSTEM DYSFUNCTIONS
CNS

CVA, peripheral neuropathy, retinopathy

HEART

silent MI, CAD, PVD, arrhythmias,
autonomic neuropathy (resting tachycardia, orthostatic hypotension)

GI

gastroparesis (full stomach?)

KIDNEY

chronic renal failure
neurogenic bladder (urosepsis?)

OB/GYN

fetal hypoglycemia, fetal death from placenta insufficiency, macrosomia

OTHER

infection, poor wound healing,
atlanto-occipital joint stiffness (difficult airway?)

MANAGEMENT
PRE-OP

Evaluate other organ dysfunctions (silent MI, renal failure, etc.).
Rule out ketoacidosis.(*No elective surgery should be done.*)
Premedicate with a H_2 blocker and Reglan.
On the day of surgery, check [glucose], start D5 ½NS, and
administer the ½ dose insulin/no oral hypoglycemic agent.

INTRA-OP

Monitor [glucose] q1h.
Maintain [glucose] at 100-200 mg/dL.
Start Regular insulin IV at 1 unit/h per 150 mg/dL glucose if uncontrolled.
Avoid hypoglycemia (<50 mg/dL):
Sympathetic activation (hypertension, tachycardia, diaphoresis)
CNS injury (headache, N/V, seizures, coma.)
Monitor [K^+], pH, [acetone].

POST-OP

Monitor [glucose].

DIABETIC KETOACIDOSIS (DKA)

PRECIPITATING FACTORS
Stress:
> MI, infection, sepsis, dehydration,
> surgery, trauma, pregnancy

Drugs:
> steroids, glucagon, $beta_2$ agonists

COMPLICATIONS
metabolic acidosis
dehydration/hypovolemia
hypokalemia

MANAGEMENT
Treat the precipitating factors.
Check ABG, electrolytes for acidosis, hypokalemia, pseudohyponatremia.
Start IV hydration and Regular insulin at 0.1 unit/kg/h (10 units/h) IV.
Supplement K^+ at <40 mEq/h IV only if good urine output is present.
Stop insulin if [glucose] < 250 mg/dL; start D5 ½NS IV.
Consider $NaHCO_3$ if pH < 7.20 or BE < -10.

HYPEROSMOLAR HYPERGLYCEMIC NONKETOTIC COMA

PRECIPITATING FACTORS
Stress:
> MI, infection, sepsis, dehydration (from impaired thirst drive in old age),
> surgery, trauma, CPB

Drugs:
> TPN, diuretics, steroids

COMPLICATIONS
dehydration/hypovolemia from diuresis with osm >300 mOsm/L & [glucose] >600 mg/dL
CNS depression from cerebral dehydration

TREATMENT
Administer insulin to lower [glucose] to 300 mg/dL (gradually to avoid cerebral edema).
Maintain IV fluid resuscitation.

HYPERTHYROIDISM

☞ *Delay the surgery until thyroid function is normal.*

Biochemical reactions, O_2 consumption, heat production are increased.
MAC is not increased (but hyperthermia increases MAC by 5%/°C).
Beta-adrenergic receptor sensitivity is increased. (up-regulation)
Affects females in 20s-40s.

Diagnosis:
    Check TFT for elevated $[T_4]$.

SIGNS & SYMPTOMS
HEART
    Tachycardia:
☞ *Avoid atropine, ketamine, pancuronium; omit epinephrine in the local anesthetics.*
    Atrial fibrillation:
☞ *Check ECG.*

AIRWAY/ LUNG
    Goiter:
☞ *Evaluate the airway with H&P, CXR, CT, flow-volume loop.*
    Muscle weakness:
☞ *Use a muscle twitch monitor.*

OTHER
    Exophthalmos:
☞ *Protect the eyes intra-op.*

TREATMENT
    Optimize thyroid function before surgery (no arrhythmia, HR <90, SBP <140 mm Hg).

DRUG	ACTION	DOSAGE/RESULT	SIDE EFFECTS
PTU (propylthiouracil)	inhibits **synthesis** of thyroid hormone	150 mg q6h/1-2 mon	bleeding from agranulocytosis
iodide	inhibits **release** of thyroid hormone	1-2 g IV/10 days	hypothyroidism from radioactivity
propranolol	inhibits **effect** of thyroid hormone	80 mg q8h/10 days	bronchospasm from beta blockade

GOITER & AIRWAY OBSTRUCTION

CAUSES
PRE-OP

☞ *Take a careful H&P; check CXR, CT, flow-volume loop*.*

Goiter
Mediastinal mass

* <u>Extrathoracic</u> variable lesion reduces the area of <u>inspiratory</u> limb.
<u>Intrathoracic</u> variable lesion reduces the area of <u>expiratory</u> limb.

POST-OP

Hematoma:

☞ *Cut the surgical suture to relieve the airway obstruction.*

Recurrent laryngeal nerve injury:

☞ *Complete vocal cord obstruction can occur if the nerve injury is bilateral.*

Laryngospasm (from hypocalcemia from hypoparathyroidism on day 1-3 post-op):

☞ *Administer CaCl₂.*

Edema:

☞ *Check for air leak around the deflated cuff before extubation.*

Tracheomalacia:

☞ *Anticipate possible airway collapse if the lesion is long-standing.*

Pneumothorax:

☞ *Check CXR.*

THYROID STORM

Signs & symptoms:
hyperthermia, tachycardia, AF, shock, CHF (similar to MH*)

Onset:
occurs intra-op or early post-op. (<24 h)

Precipitating factors:
surgery, trauma, infection, sepsis, DKA, pregnancy.

Treatment:
IV fluid, cooling, steroids,
PTU, iodide, beta blockers.

* *Unlike MH, thyroid storm often lacks severe acidosis, muscle rigidity, myoglobinuria, or CPK elevation.*

HYPOTHYROIDISM

☞ *Delay the surgery until thyroid function is close to normal.*

Biochemical reactions, O_2 consumption, heat production are decreased.
MAC is not decreased (but hypothermia decreases MAC by 5%/°C).
Usually affects female, elderly.

Diagnosis:
    Check TFT for elevated [TSH] with low [T_4] (<1 µg/dL).

SIGNS & SYMPTOMS
CNS
    lethargy from hyponatremia, hypoglycemia, hypothermia
☞ *Protect the airway.*
HEART
    hypotension, bradycardia, pericardial effusion, CHF
☞ *Consider ketamine, cortisol.*
LUNG
    hypoventilation from muscle weakness and increased sensitivity to depressants
☞ *Be cautious with sedatives.*
GI
    delayed gastric emptying
☞ *Premedicate with Reglan and a H_2 blocker.*
LIVER/KIDNEY
    slow drug metabolism
☞ *Reduce the anesthetic dosages.*

TREATMENT
    T_4 (Thyroxine or Synthroid):
        takes 10 days to be effective.
    T_3 (Levothyroxine or Triiodothyronine):
        takes 6 hours to be effective.
        MI can occur in patients with CAD.
    Cortisol

MYXEDEMA COMA

    A severe case of hypothyroidism with CHF, coma.
    Mortality is 50%.
    Treatment includes T_3, T_4, cortisol.

PHEOCHROMOCYTOMA

Pathophysiology:
   overproduction of norepinephrine (NE) & epinephrine from the tumor

Triad:
   headache, palpitation, diaphoresis

Hallmark:
   paroxysmal HTN

Diagnosis:
   urine assay for VMA, metanephrine (catecholamine metabolites)
   blood assay for catecholamines
   CT
   clonidine suppression test

MANAGEMENT
PRE-OP
Stabilize hemodynamics (Roizen, 1984):
   BP <165/90 for 48 h
   PVCs <5 for 5 min
   no ST-T changes in ECG for 2 weeks

Cardiac evaluation:
   Check ECG.
   Rule out cardiomyopathy.

Alpha blockade:
   Nasal stuffiness, orthostatic hypotension develop with alpha blockade.
   Phenoxybenzamine 50-100 mg PO qd for 2 weeks
   Prazosin avoids reflex tachycardia.

Hydration:
   to compensate for vasodilation from alpha blockade
   Hct will decrease by 5% with adequate hydration.
   Orthostatic hypotension should be >80/45.

Beta blockade:
   after alpha blockade
   after ruling out cardiomyopathy

INTRA-OP

Regional anesthesia does not block alpha-adrenergic response to catecholamines.

Establish an A-line and a PA catheter.
Deepen anesthesia before laryngoscopy.
Avoid halothane, ketamine, pancuronium, histamine releasers, droperidol, or Reglan.
Maintain SBP at 100-200 mm Hg with
phenylephrine, norepinephrine, or nitroprusside, esmolol, phentolamine.
Be vigilant for hypotension and hypoglycemia after ligation of venous drainage from
the adrenal glands.

POST-OP

Monitor hemodynamics closely.
Monitor [glucose] for possible hypoglycemia.

CARCINOID SYNDROME

serotonin, kinins, histamines

Pathophysiology:
   from massive release of the vasoactive substances from the tumor of GI tract

Diagnosis:
   urine assay for 5-OH indole-acetic acid (a serotonin metabolite)

SIGNS & SYMPTOMS
Histamine, Kallikrein:
   skin flushing, hypotension, bronchospasm

Serotonin:
   sedation (decreased MAC)
   hypertension, hyperglycemia, hypoalbuminemia,
   diarrhea, sedation

R-side heart diseases from plaque deposit:
   conduction problem (SVT)
   valve lesions (tricuspid insufficiency, pulmonic stenosis)

MANAGEMENT
PRE-OP
   IV hydration
   octreotide (a somatostatin analogue) 50 µg IV/SC
   H_1 & H_2 blockers, steroids
   Establish an A-line, CVP/PAC.

INTRA-OP
   Avoid sympathetic activation (e.g., ketamine, pancuronium).
   Avoid histamine releasers.
   Treat hypotension with IV fluid and angiotensin instead of catecholamines.

DIABETES INSIPIDUS (DI) & SYNDROME OF INAPPROPRIATE ANTIDIURETIC HORMONE SECRETION (SIADH)

ADH (Vasopressin) enhances resorption of free water in the renal collecting ducts.

	DI	SIADH

Pathophysiology	deficit of ADH:
	    lack of ADH (neurogenic)
	    insensitivity to ADH (nephrogenic)
		excess of ADH

Causes	trauma to pituitary (hypophysectomy) hypothermia, lithium, alcohol	lung CA, hypothyroidism surgery, positive pressure ventilation
Signs & Symptoms	"dehydration" hypernatremia, brain shrinkage low urine osm; high urine output	"water intoxication" hyponatremia, cerebral edema high urine osm; low urine output
Treatment	D5 ¼NS DDAVP (for neurogenic DI) Chlorpropamide (for nephrogenic DI)	NS, fluid restriction Demeclocycline

13

NEUROSURGERY & ANESTHESIA

☞ *The goal is to control intracranial pressure (ICP).*
☞ *ABC before ICP.*

CUSHING'S REFLEX
Consists of hypertension, bradycardia, irregular breathing patterns.
Implies increased ICP and impending brain herniation.

GLASGOW COMA SCALE
Scale ranges from 3 to 15:
   eye opening (1-4) + verbal response (1-5) + motor control (1-6)
Scale below 8 represents severe injury/coma:
☞ *Intubate & hyperventilate!*

HUNT & HESS CLASSIFICATION OF RUPTURED ANEURYSMS

GRADE	SIGNS &SYMPTOMS	MORTALITY
1	minimal	5%
2	HA, nuchal rigidity	10%
3	drowsiness, confusion	15%
4	stupor, hemiparesis	60%
5	coma, decerebrate rigidity	100%

BRAIN PROTECTION
Hypothermia:
   more effective than barbiturate
Barbiturate:
   good for focal ischemia, not for global ischemia (e.g., cardiac arrest)
Steroid:
   good for acute spinal cord injury, not for brain injury

CEREBRAL BLOOD FLOW (CBF) & INTRACRANIAL PRESSURE (ICP)

ICP is normally 5-15 mm Hg.

CBF is directly related to ICP.

CBF remains constant at 50 ml/100 g brain/min by autoregulation when MAP 50-150 mmHg.

The MAP of autoregulation is shifted to a higher range in patients with chronic HTN.

Autoregulation is impaired by trauma, tumor, drugs (inhalational agents, vasodilators).

CBF/ICP IS *INCREASED* BY

Hypoxemia:
> PaO_2 <50 mm Hg

Hypercarbia:
> $PaCO_2$ above 25 mm Hg at the rate of 1 ml/100 g/min per mm Hg elevation

Hypertension:
>   MAP >150 mm Hg

Hyperthermia:
>   increased $CMRO_2$

Venous congestion:
>   increased CVP by PEEP, laryngoscopy, coughing, seizures, pain,
>   extreme neck twisting, and Trendelenburg position

Drugs:
> N_2O/inhalational agents   (MAC <1 and low $PaCO_2$ blunt the increase.)
>   ketamine
>   vasodilators/histamine releasers
>   succinylcholine   (Defasciculation with a nondepolarizer blunts the increase.)

CBF/ICP IS *DECREASED* BY

Hypocarbia:
> $PaCO_2$ down to 25 mm Hg at the rate of 1 ml/100 g/min per mm Hg reduction

Hypotension:
>   MAP <50 mm Hg   (Cerebral perfusion is also decreased.)

Hypothermia
>   decreased $CMRO_2$

Venous drainage:
>   reverse Trendelenburg position

CSF drainage:
>   lumbar puncture   *(Beware of possible brain herniation.)*

Drugs:
>   barbiturates, etomidate, narcotics, benzodiazepines
>   steroids   *(Use for tumor edema; peak in 12-36 h.)*
>   mannitol   *(Do not use with CHF or disrupted BBB.)*
>   furosemide

CEREBRAL VASCULAR ACCIDENT (CVA)

☞ *Maintain cerebral perfusion (CPP = MAP − ICP).*
☞ *Avoid hyperglycemia, hypovolemia, hypotonia (e.g., D5 ½NS).*
☞ *Maintain hypothermia.*
☞ *Delay elective surgical procedures for 6 months.*

CEREBRAL HEMORRHAGE

Epidural hematoma:
  Associated with loss of consciousness (LOC), skull fracture.
  Signs & symptoms develop in hours.
  arterial (middle meningeal artery)

Subdural hematoma:
  Associated with headache (HA), blunt trauma.
  Signs & symptoms may develop in days.
  venous

Subarachnoid hemorrhage ("ruptured aneurysm"):
  Associated with HA, mental status change, coma, ECG changes, vasospasm, rebleeding.
  Signs & symptoms usually develop suddenly.
  Risk factors include size >10 mm, HTN, anticoagulation.
  Control <u>BP</u> with nitroprusside, esmolol, trimethaphan, carotid compression.
  Treat <u>vasospasm</u> with nimodipine, IV fluid.

Intracerebral hemorrhage (AV malformation):
  Associated with seizures.
  Signs & symptoms often develop slowly.

CEREBRAL ISCHEMIA

Cerebral thrombosis:
  Risk factors include vascular lesions (smoking, DM).

Cerebral embolism:
  Risk factors include AF, valve lesions, mural thrombus, MI, TIA, CPB.

SITTING CRANIOTOMY & VENOUS AIR EMBOLISM

Venous air embolism can precipitate cardiopulmonary collapse.

A precordial Doppler is a very sensitive detector for it.

A multi-orificed CVP line should be inserted for potential aspiration of air.

DETECTION

(in order of decreasing sensitivity)

1. TEE
2. Precordial Doppler
3. Hypoxia, N_2 on mass spectrometry
4. Sudden decrease in $PECO_2$; increase in $PaCO_2$, CVP, PAP
5. Tachycardia, ECG changes, hypotension
6. "Mill wheel" murmur by the esophageal stethoscope (late sign)

MANAGEMENT

Stop further air entry:

Flood the surgical field with fluid.

Turn off N_2O; administer 100% O_2.

Compress the jugular vein.

Attempt to remove the air lock:

Aspirate air through the multi-orificed CVP line.

Maintain the intracardiac blood flow:

Increase CVP with IV fluid, PEEP.

Support hemodynamics with vasopressers.

Position the patient to Trendelenburg & left lateral decubitus
to keep the intracardiac outflow tract open.

OTHER COMPLICATIONS OF SITTING POSITION

Paradoxical embolism (R to L):

Risk factors include cardiac septal defects, ventriculoatrial shunt, pulmonary HTN, PEEP,

Hemodynamic instability:

from decreased CO; increased SVR

from cranial nerve stimulation

☞ *Avoid in patients with cardiac or cerebral diseases.*

Neurological injury:

spinal cord ischemia from hyperflexion of the neck

sciatic nerve injury from hyperextension of the knees

14

LUNG PROBLEMS

PHYSIOLOGY & DEFINITIONS

PULMONARY PARAMETERS

	FORMULA	RANGE	SIGNIFICANCE
PAO_2	$(760-47)FIO_2 - PaCO_2/0.8$	FIO_2 (%) $\times$ 5 mm Hg	alveolar O_2 tension
$A\text{-}aDO_2$	$PAO_2 - PaO_2$	<20 mm Hg with FIO_2 21% (RA) >350 mm Hg with FIO_2 100% needs intubation	alveolar-arterial O_2 gradient monitors shunt oxygenation (PO_2) efficiency
a/A	PaO_2/PAO_2	>0.75	monitors shunt compensated for changes in FIO_2
Qs/Qt	(Cc – Ca)/(Cc – Cv)	<0.05	shunt fraction
V_D/V_T	$(PaCO_2 - PECO_2)/PaCO_2$	<0.3 >0.6 needs intubation	monitors dead space ventilation (PCO_2) efficiency
V/Q	MV/CO	0.8	ventilation/perfusion match efficiency of gas exchange

ACUTE RESPIRATORY FAILURE

SHUNT
perfusion without ventilation (e.g., pneumothorax)
normal anatomic shunt from bronchial, pleural, and Thebesian veins
makes up 3% of CO
increasing FIO_2 does not improve oxygenation
expressed by A-a gradient, venous admixture

DEAD SPACE
ventilation without perfusion (e.g., PE)
normal physiologic dead space by anatomic and alveolar components
makes up at 2 ml/kg
affected by age, height, posture, pulmonary aberrations (from pathology, anesthesia)
expressed by V_D/V_T

CRITERIA FOR ACUTE RESPIRATORY FAILURE
☞ *Check PO_2, PCO_2, strength.*

Hypoxemia:
   PO_2 <60 mm Hg on FIO_2 60% (or A-a gradient >350 mm Hg on FIO_2 100%)
Hypoventilation:
   PCO_2 >50 mm Hg except in COPD (or V_D/V_T >0.6)
Abnormal respiratory mechanics:
   RR >30, VC <15 ml/kg, negative inspiratory force <-20 cm H_2O

POSITIVE END-EXPIRATORY PRESSURE (PEEP)
For PaO_2 <60 mm Hg on FIO_2 >60%.
Increases FRC; decreases shunting.
Decreases venous return and CO.
May cause pneumothorax.

PULMONARY FUNCTION TEST (PFT)

WHAT IS IT?

It measures lung volumes, gas flow, diffusion capacity.

In specific terms it refers to spirometry with FEV_1, $FEV_{25-75\%}$, FVC, MBC, etc.

Its predicted values depend on age, sex, height.

It requires patient cooperation (children usually over 6 years old).

WHO NEED IT?

Patients with the risks of perioperative respiratory failure or complications:

pulmonary diseases (COPD, restrictive lung diseases including neuromuscular diseases)

old age (over 60)

obesity

heavy smoking

procedures involving thorax, upper abdomen

WHY DO YOU NEED IT?

To establish the patients' baseline pulmonary reserve:

may be useful for weaning from mechanical ventilation

To see if the pulmonary pathology is reversible with pre-op treatment:

e.g., >15% airflow improvement in bronchial asthma treated with bronchodilators

To identify and plan for perioperative pulmonary complications.

LUNG VOLUMES

FUNCTIONAL RESIDUAL CAPACITY (FRC)

Represents the lung volume at the end of a normal expiration.

FRC is decreased with obesity, pregnancy, ascites, GA, supine position, neonates.

FRC represents pulmonary reserve.

CLOSING CAPACITY (CC)

Represents the lung volume at which small airways begin to collapse.

CC is increased with smoking, COPD, upper abdominal surgery, age >60.

CC equals to FRC in <u>supine</u> position at age <u>44</u> and in <u>standing</u> position at age <u>66.</u>

OBSTRUCTIVE LUNG DISEASES

Work of breathing is increased.
Lung volumes (RV, FRC, TLC) are increased.
FEV_1 is decreased.
FEV_1/VC ratio is also decreased.

ASTHMA

hyperactive, reversible, chronic inflammatory airway
(increased edema, permeability, secretion)

☞ *Avoid ETT; consider regional or mask inhalation techniques.*

MANAGEMENT
PRE-OP
H&P:
> Identify precipitating factors, treatment response, prior history of intubation/steroid use.
> Check for wheezing, cough, dyspnea.

Lab:
> Check CBC for increased eosinophil count.
> Check CXR for infection/air trapping.
> Consider ABG/PFT.
> (FEV_1 >50% with no symptoms; <35% with severe disease; <25% with CO_2 retention)

Optimization:
> Administer bronchodilators, IV hydration, antibiotics.
> Repeat ABG/PFT.

Premedication:
> H_2 blockers also block bronchodilation against H_1 mediated bronchoconstriction.
> Anticholinergics can produce viscous secretions.
> Consider steroid if the patient was treated within the past year for over 1 week.

INTRA-OP
> Intubate deep. (Suppress airway reflex with lidocaine, ketamine, inhalational agents.)
> Avoid histamine releasers (MSO_4, curare).
> Avoid halothane if patient is on beta agonists or aminophylline.
> Heat & humidify the inspired gas.
> Maintain adequate hydration.
> Use a low respiratory rate for ventilation to avoid air trapping.
> Extubate deep or wide awake.

BRONCHOSPASM

☞ *Wheezing is not always caused by bronchospasm; rule out other causes of wheezing.*

CAUSES OF WHEEZING
Airway:
ETT obstruction/foreign body
endobronchial intubation/stimulation of carina

Lung:
aspiration, pulmonary embolism, pneumothorax, *bronchospasm*

Heart:
pulmonary edema

SIGNS & SYMPTOMS
O_2 desaturation   (decreased gas exchange)
wheezing   (decreased gas flow)
increased PIP   (decreased lung compliance)

TREATMENT
Deepen the anesthesia with an inhalational agent/IV agents.

Administer a beta$_2$ agonist via ETT:
Albuterol (Proventil, Ventolin), Metaproterenol (Alupent): 2-4 puffs
Terbutaline (Brethine): 0.25 mg SC q15min × 3 prn
It increases [cAMP] by stimulating the adenyl cyclase.

Administer aminophylline:
Loading dose: 5 mg/kg IV over 20 min.
Maintenance: 0.5 mg/kg/h IV
It increases [cAMP] by inhibiting phosphodiesterase.
It can cause seizures, arrhythmias (especially with halothane or epinephrine).

Administer beta adrenergic agonists:
Epinephrine: 0.3 ml of 1:1,000 SC q15 min × 3 prn
Racemic epinephrine: 0.5 ml in 3 ml NS via nebulizer
Isoproterenol: 0.1 μg/min IV

☞ *Check ABG.*

Steroids, cromolyn sodium, Atrovent (ipratropium bromide) and antihistamines
are not generally useful for acute treatment because of their delayed onset.

CHRONIC OBSTRUCTIVE PULMONARY DISEASE (COPD)
CHRONIC BRONCHITIS & EMPHYSEMA

MANAGEMENT
PRE-OP
Check ABG/PFT:

PCO_2 >50 mm Hg, FEV_1/VC <50% indicate high risks for post-op respiratory failure.

Check CXR for RVH, bullae or infection.

Check sputum for infection.

Check for signs of pulmonary HTN, cor pulmonale (RVH, JVD, edema).

Optimize pulmonary status:

hydration, antibiotics, bronchodilators, nutrition

Stop smoking:

to decrease carboxyhemoglobin level and shift $Hb-O_2$ curve to the right (in hours)

to restore mucocilliary function and decrease secretions (in months)

to restore immune function (in months)

INTRA-OP
Consider regional techniques, but avoid motor blockade above T6

to preserve expiratory reserve volume (cough reflex).

Be careful if using narcotics for sedation (blunted respiratory drive to increased PCO_2).

Consider rupture of bullae, especially with N_2O (tension pneumothorax?).

Heat & humidify the inspiratory gas.

Maintain hydration.

Set a large TV and a slow RR to avoid air trapping.

POST-OP
Clear the secretions & avoid atelectasis:

epidural/intrathecal opioids or nerve blocks for post-op pain

chest PT

incentive spirometry

RESTRICTIVE LUNG DISEASES

Lung compliance and diffusion capacity are decreased.
Lung volumes (FRC, RV, TLC) are decreased.
Both FEV_1 and VC are decreased.
FEV_1/VC ratio remains unchanged.

CAUSES

INTRINSIC (LUNG)
ACUTE
> Pulmonary edema:
>> from fluid overload (CHF from MI, negative pressure)
>> from leaky capillary vessels (ARDS from aspiration, fat embolism, trauma/burn)

CHRONIC
> Pulmonary fibrosis:
>> sarcoidosis, SLE
>> bleomycin, radiation therapy

EXTRINSIC (CHEST WALL)
ACUTE
> Normal compliance:
>> flail chest, spinal cord injury

> Decreased compliance:
>> pneumothorax, hemothorax, pleural effusion

CHRONIC
> Normal compliance:
>> neuromuscular diseases (myasthenia gravis, muscular dystrophy, multiple sclerosis)

> Decreased compliance:
>> obesity, ascites, pregnancy, kyphoscoliosis, mediastinal mass

ASPIRATION PNEUMONITIS

Mortality is increased with pH <2.5 and volume >25 ml.
Characterized by hypoxemia, bronchospasm and decreased lung compliance.
CXR does not reveal RLL or RML infiltrates for first 8-12 hours.

Treatment includes 100% O_2, mechanical ventilation with PEEP, and bronchodilators.
Bronchoscopy should be performed.
Irrigation with NS is not recommended.
Prophylactic antibiotics and steroids are not recommended.

ANTERIOR MEDIASTINAL MASS
☞ *Keep the patient spontaneously breathing.*
☞ *Be prepared to manage complete airway obstruction upon induction of general anesthesia!*

FLOW-VOLUME LOOP
Extrathoracic variable lesion reduces the area of inspiratory limb.
Intrathoracic variable lesion reduces the area of expiratory limb.

CAUSES
5 Ts: **T**hyroid, **T**hymoma, **T**eratoma, **T**horacic aneurysm, **T**errible lymphoma

MANAGEMENT
PRE-OP
Check CXR, CT, flow-volume loop, and echocardiogram to evaluate the lesion.
Consider radiation therapy to shrink the mass lesion.
Establish IV access in the lower extremity if SVC syndrome is present.
Be prepared for emergency rigid bronchoscopy and/or CPB.
Avoid premedication with respiratory depressants.

INTRA-OP
Maintain spontaneous respiration:
    inhalational induction for a child
    awake fiberoptic intubation for an adult
If acute airway obstruction occurs, turn the patient to side or prone position
to relieve the obstruction.
If failed, establish an airway by emergency rigid bronchoscopy.
If failed, start CPB.

POST-OP
Do not extubate the patient until it is certain that airway collapse will not occur.
Beware of potential pneumothorax and hemorrhage.

ONE-LUNG VENTILATION & THORACOTOMY

<u>Nondependent</u> lung refers to <u>nonventilated</u> lung.

  <u>Dependent</u> lung refers to   <u>ventilated</u> lung.

Keep MV unchanged. (CO_2 does not build up due to high solubility.)

Hypoxic pulmonary vasoconstriction (HPV) reduces V/Q mismatch.

DOUBLE-LUMEN TUBE

INDICATIONS

ABSOLUTE

  Isolation of blood, pus, gas:

    hemorrhage, abscess, lavage, cyst, bronchopleural fistula

RELATIVE

  Exposure of surgical sites:

    pneumonectomy, upper lobectomy, thoracic aortic aneurysm
    esophageal surgery

ROBERTSHAW-TYPE DOUBLE-LUMEN TUBE

  Size:

        28 FR for child (age 10-12)
      35, 37 FR for female
      39, 41 FR for male

      $FR = 6 \times (ID\ in\ mm) + 3$

  Left vs. Right bronchial-sided tube:

    A **right** bronchial-sided tube is preferred for **left**   main bronchus lesions.
    A **left**   bronchial-sided tube is preferred for **right** main bronchus lesions.
    A **left**   bronchial-sided tube is preferred for **left**   lung ventilation.
    A *left*   bronchial-sided tube is preferred for **right** lung ventilation (not to miss
    the right upper lobe ventilation).

PNEUMONECTOMY & PRE-OP EVALUATION

Pneumonectomy is contraindicated if... (Benumof, 1987)

1. **TOTAL** LUNG STUDY shows
   ABG: PCO_2 >50 mm Hg
   PFT: FEV_1 <50% (< 2 L),
      MBC <50%,
      RV/TLC >50% of predicted

2. **SPLIT** LUNG STUDY USING XENON V/Q SCAN shows
   V/Q: blood flow to the diseased lung >70%
      FEV_1 of the healthy lung <0.8 L

3. **POST-OP** SIMULATION STUDY USING PA OCCLUSION METHOD shows
   ABG: PCO_2 >60 mm Hg,
      PaO_2 <40 mm Hg
   PAC: MPAP >40 mm Hg

HYPOXEMIA & ONE-LUNG VENTILATION

CAUSES

V/Q mismatch from shunting via:

GENERAL ANESTHESIA

V: Decreases FRC; causes atelectasis and shunting.

Q: Hypoxic pulmonary vasoconstriction (HPV) is impaired by:

> Drugs (vasodilators, vasoconstrictors, calcium channel blockers, beta$_2$ agonists)
> N_2O
> PEEP, pulmonary HTN, hypothermia, hypocarbia

MUSCLE RELAXATION & MECHANICAL VENTILATION

V: Abdominal content against diaphragm impairs ventilation of lower portion of the lung.

Q: Gravity favors perfusion of lower portion of the lung.

LATERAL DECUBITUS POSITION

Compression of the dependent lung by the mediastinum

V: Causes hypoventilation of the dependent lung.

Q: Decreases venous return and CO.

OPEN CHEST

Obliteration of the intrathoracic negative pressure

V: Causes the lungs to collapse.

Q: Decreases venous return and CO.

ONE-LUNG VENTILATION

V: Collapsed lung is not ventilated.

Q: But it is still perfused.

TREATMENT

1. Administer 100% O_2.
2. Apply CPAP 5-10 cm H_2O to the nondependent lung.
3. Apply PEEP 5-10 cm H_2O to the dependent lung.
4. Inflate the nondependent lung every 5-10 minutes.
5. Increase CO.
6. Clamp the PA of the nondependent lung.
7. Ventilate both lungs.

15

HEART PROBLEMS

The goal is to balance **O$_2$ demand** and **supply** to heart.

PULMONARY ARTERY CATHETER (PAC)

INDICATIONS
"to optimize the filling pressure and to maximize the cardiac output..."

LV dysfunction:
CHF, valvular heart diseases, recent MI, severe cardiac dysfunction (unstable angina)

Pulmonary HTN:
severe COPD, massive PE, severe acute pulmonary dysfunction (ARDS)

Hemodynamic instability:
major fluid shift, aortic cross-clamping, shock, inotrope infusion

CONTRAINDICATIONS (relative)
Conduction defect:
complete LBBB, WPW syndrome

Valvular defect:
Ebstein's malformation, mechanical heart valve

PARAMETERS MEASURED
CO (Thermodilutional change of the injectate temperature is inversely proportional to CO.)
CVP/PCWP
PvO$_2$
PAP
Blood temperature

PARAMETERS DERIVED
SVR/PVR
SV
CI

PULMONARY ARTERY RUPTURE
Mortality is about 50%.

Risk factors:
pulmonary HTN
coagulopathy
catheter migration
"overwedging"

Signs & symptoms:
hemoptysis
chest pain
hypoxemia

Management:
Secure the airway with a double-lumen tube.
Do not remove the PAC.
Keep the bleeding side down.
Consider NTG to reduce PAP.

PHYSIOLOGY & DEFINITIONS

HEMODYNAMIC PARAMETERS

	FORMULAS	RANGE	COMMENTS
MAP	DBP + (SBP − DBP)/3	70-110 mm Hg	pulse pressure = SBP − DBP
MPAP	DPAP + (SPAP − DPAP)/3	10-20 mm Hg	MPAP>35mm Hg can cause RV failure. Dicrotic notch represents pulmonic valve closure.
CVP	**a wave:** atrial contraction **c wave:** valve into atrium **x descent:** atrial relaxation **v wave:** atrial filling **y descent:** ventricular filling	0-10 mm Hg	does not reflect volume status accurately in patients with LV dysfunction, valvular heart diseases, pulmonary HTN (COPD, edema, PE) or HR > 120.
PCWP or wedge	Check at the end of expiration: Read the <u>high</u> side of tracing in <u>spontaneous</u> ventilation. Read the <u>low</u> side of tracing in <u>mechanical</u> ventilation.	5-15 mm Hg	preload (PCWP = LVEDP = LVEDV) PCWP > LVEDP with MS, MR and increased intrathoracic, intrapulmonary pressure PCWP < LVEDP with AS, AR and noncompliant LV (LVEDP >25 mmHg)
CO	SV × HR	3-8 L/min	SV (normally 60-100): determined by preload, afterload, contractility, wall motion, valvular function.
CI	CO/BSA	2.5-5 L/m^2	CO compensated for body size
EF	(EDV − ESV)/EDV	> 55%	contractility
SVR	[(MAP − CVP)/CO] × 80	800-1,600	afterload
CaO$_2$	1.34Hb x SaO$_2$ + 0.003 PaO$_2$	20 ml/dL	O$_2$ content
DO$_2$	CaO$_2$ × CO	1,000 ml/min	O$_2$ delivery
VO$_2$	C(a-v)O$_2$ × CO	250 ml/min	O$_2$ consumption could be low due to unloading problems (met-Hb, carbon monoxide poisoning, cyanide toxicity, hypothermia, alkalosis) high due to increased consumption (sepsis, shivering, fever)

	FORMULAS	RANGE	COMMENTS
SvO_2 PvO_2	$SaO_2 - VO_2/(Hb \times CO)$	70% 40 mm Hg	Mixed venous O_2 saturation/tension monitors the balance between tissue O_2 delivery & consumption. <u>low</u> with low O_2 delivery (low CO) or high consumption (shivering, sepsis); <u>high</u> with high CO or unloading problems or wedged catheter
CPP	DBP – LVEDP (= PCWP)	60 mm Hg	coronary perfusion pressure

DETERMINANTS OF STROKE VOLUME (SV)

PRELOAD
Defined as the muscle fiber length prior to contraction.
Refers to the amount of blood in the left ventricle to be pumped out (LVEDV).
Estimated by PCWP (= LVEDP = LVEDV).
Depends on venous return, HR, rhythm.
Directly proportional to CO within the Starling's law

AFTERLOAD
Defined as the ventricular wall tension during contraction.
Refers to the resistance against which the left ventricle must pump.
Estimated by SVR = (MAP – CVP)/CO × 80 (normally 800-1,600 dynes/sec/cm^5).
Depends on SVR, contractile force of the ventricle, compliance of the aorta.
Inversely proportional to CO (e.g., CHF, aortic-cross clamping).

CONTRACTILITY
Defined as the rate of muscle fiber shortening (dP/dt, Vmax).
Refers to the intrinsic pumping force.
Estimated by EF = (EDV – ESV)/EDV (normally >55%).
Depends on intracellular $[Ca^{++}]$ which can be mediated by
beta$_1$ receptor, Na$^+$-K$^+$ ATPase, cAMP.
Directly proportional to CO except in MVP, IHSS, tet-spell.

MYOCARDIAL ISCHEMIA (MI)

MI occurs when myocardial O_2 demand exceeds supply.
Associated with chest pain, hypotension, arrhythmias, ECG changes.

O_2 DEMAND
Wall tension:
    preload
    afterload
Contractility
HR

O_2 SUPPLY
Coronary blood flow:
    coronary perfusion pressure (DBP – PCWP)
    coronary perfusion time (HR)
Coronary blood O_2 content:
    Hb
    SaO_2

RISK FACTS

INCIDENCE
0.15% for patients <u>without</u> prior MI
5% for patients <u>with</u>　prior MI
16-37% for patients <u>with</u>　prior MI, who undergo surgery within 6 months of MI

MORTALITY
30% for patients <u>without</u> prior MI
>50% for patients <u>with</u>　prior MI

RISKS FOR CAD
male
old age
HTN
smoking
hypercholesterolemia
DM
obesity
a sedentary lifestyle
family history

GOLDMAN'S CRITERIA (9) for perioperative risks for MI (1977)*
(in order of decreasing Multifactorial Index Score)

CHF/ LV DYSFUNCTION
   JVD/S3

ISCHEMIA
   MI <6 months ago
   PVC >5/min.

ARRHYTHMIA
   rhythm other than NSR

GENERAL CONDITION
   age >70
   emergency
   intrathoracic/intraperitoneal/aortic surgery
   AS
   general poor condition

☞ *Note that HTN and angina are not risk factors according to the study.*
* The study has several limitations in terms of sample size, lack of uniform criteria for detecting the risk factors/complications.

RISKS FOR REINFARCTION
   Rate of Reinfarction and the Post-MI Time at which the surgery was performed.

POST MI MONTHS	Tarhan et al. (1972)	Rao et al. (1983)*
under 3 months	37%	5.7%
under 6 months	16%	2.3%
over 6 months	5%	1.7%

*with aggressive invasive hemodynamic monitoring and therapy

RISKS FOR LV FAILURE
   EF <40%
   PCWP >18 mm Hg
   CI <2.0 L/min/m²
   dyskinesis

PRE-OP TESTS
☞ *Evaluate for ischemia, LV dysfunction, arrhythmias.*

THALLIUM STRESS TEST
Thallium is a radioactive K^+ analogue used to exclude ischemic areas ("cold spots").

Exercise:
treadmill

Resting:
Dipyridamole (Persantine) causes coronary steal by vasodilation and decreases O_2 supply.
Dobutamine increases contractility and increases O_2 demand.

CORONARY ANGIOGRAPHY
Indicated for *unstable angina*:
changes in frequency, intensity, precipitating events within the past 60 days
chest pain at rest
new onset

Three-vessel disease and left main coronary lesion carry a high risk for perioperative MI;
CABG or angioplasty should be considered before the surgical procedure.

The test procedure carries 0.1% mortality rate.

ECHOCARDIOGRAPHY
Evaluates chamber size, filling, valves, wall motion, EF.

Advantages:
noninvasive, inexpensive

Disadvantages:
requires constant visual monitoring

HOLTER ECG
Identifies silent ischemic episodes, arrhythmias.

Advantages:
very specific; the negative result correlates well clinically

Disadvantages:
does not evaluate ischemic area or LV function

INTRA-OP DIAGNOSIS
(in order of decreasing sensitivity)

1. TEE: wall motion abnormalities
2. PAC: increased wedge pressure (unreliable)
    a large *a* wave (>15 mm Hg) from stiffening of LV from ischemia
    a large *v* wave on wedge tracing of MR caused by papillary muscles dysfunction
3. ECG: ST changes, PVCs
    Leads II + V_5 detect 95% of ischemic episodes.
4. PAC: decreased CO (TEE: decreased EF)

70% of MI episodes are silent.
50% of MI episodes occur without hemodynamic changes.

TREATMENT

Decrease O_2 DEMAND.
Decrease **preload**:
    NTG, diuretics

Decrease **afterload**:
    NTG, nitroprusside

Decrease **contractility**:
    beta blockers, Ca^{++} channel blockers, halothane

Decrease **HR**:
    esmolol

Increase O_2 SUPPLY.
Increase **coronary blood flow**:
    Increase coronary perfusion pressure:
        NTG and Ca^{++} channel blockers for coronary vasodilation
    Increase coronary perfusion time:
        Treat tachycardia with esmolol.

Increase coronary blood **O_2 content**:
    Increase Hb:
        Treat anemia; keep Hct >30%.
    Increase SaO_2:
        Treat hypoxia; administer 100% O_2.

CONGESTIVE HEART FAILURE (CHF)

☞ *Delay elective surgical procedures if possible as the mortality rate is consistently high.*
☞ *Avoid depressing contractility further; consider etomidate, narcotics and epidural technique.*

RISKS FOR LV FAILURE
EF <40%
PCWP >18 mm Hg
CI <2.0 L/min/m^2
dyskinesis

PATHOPHYSIOLOGY
Decreased CO results in **hypotension** and **pulmonary edema**, which in turn result in
metabolic acidosis from tissue hypoperfusion and tissue hypoxia (SvO_2 <60%).
LVH, Na$^+$ retention, tachycardia and peripheral **vasoconstriction** occur
to compensate for decreased CO via sympathetic activation of the autonomic nerve system.

PATHOPHYSIOLOGY	CAUSES	SIGNS & SYMPTOMS	TREATMENT
PRELOAD overload	**fluid overload** L to R shunt (VSD, ASD, PDA)	high LVEDP (PCWP) pulmonary edema JVD, pedal edema	**diuretics** fluid restriction NTG
AFTERLOAD overload	**vasoconstriction** HTN	high SVR cold, clammy skin metabolic acidosis	**vasodilators** nitroprusside amrinone
CONTRACTILITY deficit	**LV pump failure** cardiomyopathy MI valve dysfunction	low SV (EF <40%) hypotension, S3 oliguria	ketamine pure narcotics **inotropes** digoxin dopamine dobutamine amrinone IABP

COR PULMONALE (RV FAILURE)

PATHOPHYSIOLOGY
RV afterload overload

CAUSES
LV failure, pulmonary HTN (COPD, morbid obesity), massive PE

SIGNS & SYMPTOMS
Physical exam:
JVD, S3, hepatojugular reflux, pedal edema

ECG:
RAD/RBBB/RVH
large P waves, ST-T changes on the inferior leads

MANAGEMENT
Decrease PVR:
Avoid hypoxemia, hypercarbia, acidosis.
Treat bronchospasm, infection from COPD.
Administer diuretics, vasodilators (NTG), nitric oxide (NO), digoxin, amrinone.
Consider anticoagulants if polycythemia is severe (Hct >55%).

HYPERTENSION (HTN)

☞ *Diastolic BP should be <110 mm Hg.*
Continue all the cardiac medications except diuretics on the day of surgery.
The autoregulation curve for the cerebral perfusion is shifted to the right.

MANAGEMENT
☞ *Rule out hypoxia, hypercarbia, MI, increased ICP, hypoglycemia in acute HTN.*
☞ *Take a careful H&P.*

Evaluate for **end-organ dysfunctions** (heart, kidney, brain)
Beware of the chronic **hypovolemic** state.
Anticipate **labile hemodynamic** responses.

OONGENITAL HEART DISEASES

PULMONARY BLOOD FLOW

☞ *Blood flow to the lung depends on the balance between two resistances (PVR, SVR). The goal is to balance PVR and SVR to optimize the blood flow to the lung.*

☞ *Blood flow to the lung is <u>inversely</u> related to <u>PVR</u>. ("PVR Prevents PA flow.") Blood flow to the lung is <u>directly</u> related to <u>SVR</u>.*

☞ *Too much blood flow to the lung **(L to R shunt)** causes pulmonary congestion and **CHF**. Too little blood flow to the lung **(R to L shunt)** causes hypoxemia and **cyanosis**.*

☞ *"Left" side of the heart concerns with SVR, LA, LV. "Right" side of the heart concerns with PVR, RA, RV, PA/lung.*

FACTORS AFFECTING PVR & SVR

	PVR	SVR
To increase	hypoxia, hypercarbia, acidosis sympathetic activation (pain) N_2O*, positive pressure ventilation **"tet-spell"** (infundibular spasm)***	IV fluid, phenylephrine, ketamine**, pancuronium "Squatting" kinks femoral arteries.
To decrease	nitroglycerin, isoproterenol amrinone, nitric oxide (NO)	isoflurane, nitroprusside histamine releasers

* N_2O does not increase PVR in pediatric patients.

** Ketamine does not increase PVR in pediatric patients.

*** The infundibular spasm obstructs blood flow to the lung and causes cyanosis. It is precipitated by crying, pain; treated with halothane, beta blockers. (Reduce contractility.)

L TO R SHUNT
VSD, ASD, PDA

PATHOPHYSIOLOGY
too much blood flow to the lung (CHF, pulmonary congestion, pneumonia)

INDUCTION RATE
slow with IV agents; (fast with inhalational agents)*
"The more blood goes to the lung, the less IV drug goes to the brain."

MANAGEMENT

Decrease PA flow:	Increase PVR.	Decrease SVR.
Reduce L to R shunt.	Hyperinflate the lung with positive pressure ventilation. Avoid hyperventilation.	Avoid fluid overload. Maintain contractility. *isoflurane, nitroprusside, MSO$_4$*

*Only if CO is inadequate

R TO L SHUNT
TOF, Eisenmenger syndrome, tricuspid atresia (Ebstein's malformation), pulmonic atresia

PATHOPHYSIOLOGY
too little blood flow to the lung (hypoxemia, cyanosis, polycythemia, CVA, abscess)

INDUCTION RATE
fast with IV agents; slow with inhalational agents
"The less blood goes to the lung, the less gas goes to the brain."

TREATMENT

Increase PA flow:	Decrease PVR.	Increase SVR.
Reduce R to L shunt.	Avoid hypoxia, hypercarbia, acidosis. Avoid N$_2$O, high-pressure ventilation. Avoid sympathetic activation. (pain, crying, tet-spell) *nitroglycerin, isoproterenol, amrinone beta blockers, halothane, nitric oxide*	Avoid dehydration. Avoid histamine releasers. *ketamine, pancuronium, phenylephrine*

CARDIAC TAMPONADE

PATHOPHYSIOLOGY
Obstruction of the diastolic filling of heart, resulting in decreased SV, CO, and hypotension.

CAUSES
Blood:
> trauma, post-cardiac surgery, coagulopathy

Pericardial effusion:
> uremia, rheumatoid arthritis, SLE, radiation therapy, TB, viral infection, MI (Dressler)

SIGNS & SYMPTOMS
chest pain upon inspiration, friction rub, fever

Signs of heart failure:
> hypotension, tachycardia, orthopnea

Beck's triad:
> hypotension, JVD, distant heart sounds

Kussmaul's sign:
> JVD with inspiration from RV failure

Pulses paradoxus:
> >10 mm Hg decrease in SBP with inspiration

Electrical alternans:
> various QRS sizes

ECG:
> low voltage, ST T changes

Equalization of diastolic pressures (at 20 mm Hg):
> CVP = DPAP = PCWP

DIAGNOSIS
Echocardiography is the key tool for diagnosis.
Tamponade can occur at 100 ml accumulation.
CXR does not show until 250 ml accumulation.

MANAGEMENT

☞ *Perform pericardiocentesis under local anesthesia if severe and unstable.*

☞ *Avoid muscle relaxation or positive pressure ventilation.*

☞ *Maintain "**fast, full, tight, hard**." **

HR:
> *fast* (CO depends on HR as SV is low.)

Preload:
> *full* (Maintain cardiac filling with IV fluid.)

Afterload:
> *tight* (Maintain SVR high to maintain BP.)

Contractility:
> *hard* (Maintain forward flow with contractility.)

*Since SVR = (MAP − CVP)/CO,
then   MAP = SVR × CO + CVP
= SVR × (SV × HR) + CVP

Accordingly, if SV is low, CO and MAP will decrease;
in order to maintain MAP and CO, SVR, HR and CVP must remain high.

ARRHYTHMIAS

☞ Check ABC.
☞ Check ABG, electrolytes, temperature, drugs.

ECG

Reveals HR, rhythm, old MI, hypertrophy, electrolyte abnormality.
Resting ECG maybe normal in 50% of the patients with CAD.

LEADS	REGION	CORONARY ARTERY
II, III, AVF	inferior wall	right
I, AVL, V_{4-6}	lateral wall	left circumflex
V_{1-3}	anteroseptal wall	left anterior descending

The modified-V_5 lead allows the anterior wall to be monitored using 3 leads.

CAUSES OF ST SEGMENT CHANGES
ST segment elevation:
  transmural ischemia (Q wave)
  Prinzmetal's angina, cardiac contusion, pericarditis
  hyperkalemia, hypothermia
  digoxin

ST segment depression:
  subendocardial ischemia (non-Q wave)
  LBBB, PE, CNS injuries
  hypokalemia
  digoxin

SUPRAVENTRICULAR ARRHYTHMIAS

CAUSES
Heart:
>> MI, valvular diseases (AS, MS, MVP, IHSS), pericarditis
>> WPW syndrome

Lung:
>> pulmonary diseases (hypoxia, hypercarbia)

Metabolic:
>> pH/electrolyte abnormalities
>> hyperthyroidism, fever

Pharmacologic:
>> digoxin

SUPRAVENTRICULAR TACHYCARDIA (SVT)
TREATMENT
Vagal maneuvers:
>> carotid sinus massage, Valsalva maneuvers

Drugs:
>> adenosine, verapamil, esmolol, digoxin

Cardioversion:
>> 50-360 J synchronized

Atrial pacing

ATRIAL FIBRILLATION (AF)
☞ *Beware of systemic embolism; anticoagulate.*

TREATMENT
Drugs:
>> verapamil, esmolol, digoxin   (for rate control)
>> quinidine, procainamide   (for chemical conversion)

Cardioversion:
>> 100-360 J synchronized

ATRIAL FLUTTER
☞ *Vagal maneuvers is ineffective as the reentry does not pass through the AV node.*

TREATMENT
Drugs:
> verapamil, esmolol, digoxin
> quinidine, procainamide

Cardioversion:
> 50-360 J synchronized

WOLF-PARKINSON-WHITE (WPW) SYNDROME
Pathophysiology:
> An accessory pathway bypasses the AV node (pre-excitation syndrome).

Diagnostic feature:
> delta-wave, shortened PR interval

TREATMENT
☞ *Avoid sympathetic activation or hypovolemia.*

Drugs:
> adenosine, procainamide, lidocaine
☞ *Avoid digoxin, verapamil.*

Cardioversion

VENTRICULAR ARRHYTHMIAS

CAUSES
Sympathetic:
hypoxia, **hypercarbia**, pain, light anesthesia

HEART:
MI from **hypotension**, **hypertension**;
mechanical stimulation of heart

Metabolic:
hypokalemia, hypomagnesemia

Pharmacologic:
digoxin, alcohol, caffeine, cocaine, epinephrine, aminophylline

PREMATURE VENTRICULAR CONTRACTION (PVC)
INDICATIONS FOR LIDOCAINE
1. New PVCs with MI
2. Couplets
3. Multifocal
4. >6/minute
5. "R on T" phenomenon

TREATMENT
☞ *Check & support ABC.*

Drugs:
lidocaine, procainamide, bretylium

VENTRICULAR TACHYCARDIA (VT)
TREATMENT
Drugs:
lidocaine, bretylium, procainamide

Cardioversion:
200, 300, 360 J (without pulse)
100, 200, 360 J synchronized (with pulse)

Digoxin-induced Ventricular Tachycardia
TREATMENT

☞ *Do not Cardiovert.*

Drugs:
   phenytoin (1 g IV slowly), KCl, lidocaine, atropine
   Digibind (antibody)

Torsades de Pointes
Diagnostic features:
   changing QRS axis, prolonged QT interval

TREATMENT
   Drugs:
      $MgSO_4$, KCl, isoproterenol
   Pacing
☞ *Cardiovert only if absolutely necessary.*

HEART BLOCKS

FIRST-DEGREE AV BLOCK
Diagnostic feature:
> shortening of PR interval
> usually benign

SECOND-DEGREE AV BLOCK
Diagnostic feature:
> a drop of QRS

Mobitz 1 (nodal, Wenckebach):
> progressive shortening of PR interval to a drop of QRS
> usually benign

Mobitz 2 (infranodal):
> a sudden drop of QRS
> may progress to third-degree block
> pacing is indicated

THIRD-DEGREE AV BLOCK
Diagnostic feature:
> dissociation between atrial and ventricular rates

TREATMENT
> Drugs:
>> atropine, isoproterenol
> Pacemaker

RIGHT BUNDLE BRANCH BLOCK (RBBB)
Diagnostic feature:
> RSR on V_{1-3} and S on I, AVL, V_{5-6}
> usually benign

LEFT BUNDLE BRANCH BLOCK (LBBB)
Diagnostic feature:
> RR on I, AVL V_{5-6} and S on V_{1-3}
> associated with heart diseases

☞ *A complete heart block may occur during PAC insertion (1%).*

Rapid-Sequence Review of Anesthesiology

COMMON DRUGS FOR ARRHYTHMIAS

ANTIARRHYTHMICS

Name	Dose (IV)	Action	Side effects
adenosine	6, 12 mg	slows AV conduction.	bradycardia, asystole
verapamil	2.5-5 mg	slows AV conduction.	vasodilation, hypotension
esmolol	0.5 mg/kg	slows SA/AV conduction. decreases contractility.	bradycardia, CHF, bronchospasm
digoxin	0.25 mg	slows SA/AV conduction. increases contractility.	arrhythmias, AV blocks
lidocaine	1 mg/kg	slows Purkinje fibers.	hypotension sedation, seizures
procainamide	20 mg/min	slows atrial/Purkinje/ ventricular conduction.	lupus, vasodilation, hypotension, VT/VF, torsades de pointes
bretylium	5mg/kg slow 1 mg/min	increases VF threshold. depletes NE release.	HTN from initial release of NE hypotension

ALGORITHMS

☞ *Continuous ECG monitoring and IV access should be established for all patients.*

☞ *Chest compression, epinephrine, and an ETT are indicated when no pulse is present.*

☞ *Defibrillation is indicated for a rapid ventricular rate with cerebral/cardiac hypoperfusion.*

SUMMARY OF ALGORITHMS

Rhythm	Shock	ETT	Epi-nephrine	Atropine	Lidocaine	Other Antiarrhythmics	Pacing	Comments
VF/VT no pulse	200 J, 300 J, 360 J	yes	1 mg q5min		1mg/kg q8min × 3	bretylium 5, 10 mg/kg over 10 min		Repeat shock after each drug. NaHCO$_3$?
VT with pulse	If unstable, 100 J, 200 J, 360 J syn.				1mg/kg q8min × 3	procainamide 20 mg/min (max. 1000mg) bretylium 5, 10 mg/kg		precordial thump in witnessed arrest NaHCO$_3$?
Asystole		yes	1 mg q5min	1 mg q5min			yes	NaHCO$_3$?
EMD		yes	1 mg q5min					Treat the cause.* NaHCO$_3$?
Bradycardia AV blocks				1 mg × 2		isoproterenol 2-10 μg/min	yes	digoxin toxicity?
PSVT	If unstable, 100 J, 200 J, 360 J syn.					adenosine verapamil** beta blockers	yes	vagal maneuvers

* hypoxemia, acidosis, hypovolemia, cardiac tamponade, tension pneumothorax, PE
**contraindicated for WPW syndrome

CARDIOVERSION

Indicated when acute hypoperfusion of brain and heart occurs (HR > 150).
Contraindicated with *digoxin-induced* arrhythmias, hyperthyroidism, hypokalemia.

Does not harm the *fetus* in pregnancy.
Does not harm the *pacemaker* unless the current is applied directly above it.

Apply R on R, not T (R on T Phenomenon).
Elective cardioversion for AF should be performed after NPO and anticoagulation.

Complications include stroke and arrhythmias.

PACEMAKER

coded in the order of chamber *Paced*, *Sensed*, and pacer *Response,* etc. *(P before S)*.

PAC insertion can dislodge the pacemaker electrodes if <1 month old.
Beware of *microshock* during the insertion of a transvenous pacemaker.
Myopotential inhibition can occur with succinylcholine from fasciculations, and shivering.
Electrocautery (*"Bovie"*) dispersion pad should be placed far away from the pacemaker.
Defibrillation paddles should be placed far away from the pacemaker.
A *magnet* converts a pacemaker to an asynchronous mode (VOO).
MRI is contraindicated.
Pre-op tests for a pacemaker include CXR, ECG, Holter.

The following factors make pacing difficult:
   Metabolic:
       hypoxia, hypercarbia
       hyperglycemia, hypernatremia, hypokalemia
       sleep, hypothermia
   Pharmacologic:
       isoproterenol, beta blockers
       lidocaine, procainamide, quinidine
   Heart:
       MI

CARDIOPULMONARY BYPASS (CPB)

CIRCUIT

OXYGENATOR
Bubble:
> can cause cell trauma, platelet aggregation, air embolism

Membrane:
> expensive

PUMP
Roller:
> can cause cell trauma

Pulsatile:
> may provide better tissue perfusion (*controversial*)

CHECKLIST

BEFORE BYPASS
Check for adequate **anticoagulation**:
> Heparin 3 mg (300 units)/kg
> ACT >400 sec (normally 80-120 sec)

Avoid **air embolism**:
> N_2O off
> adequate reservoir/cannula priming

DURING BYPASS
Check for adequate **organ perfusion**:

MAP 50-100 mm Hg	(for brain perfusion)
PvO_2* 40-45 mm Hg	(for tissue perfusion)
urine output >1 ml/kg/h	(for kidney perfusion)
Hct 20-30%	(for overall O_2 delivery)

> *ABG Monitoring during Hypothermia*
> > *pH-stat:*
> > > *The sample is temperature-corrected*
> > > *by maintaining PCO_2 at 40 mm Hg and pH at 7.40. ("pH stays.")*
> > *α-stat:*
> > > *No CO_2 is added to compensate the gas tension changes from hypothermia.*
> > > *Some argue patient management with this mode improves overall outcome.*

COMING OFF BYPASS

Check **ABC**:

a good ETT position

bilateral breath sound present

stable hemodynamics

Hct >20%

normal ABG/electrolytes

Check the body **temperature**:

core temperature at 37°C

peripheral temperature >33°C

Check the **coagulation**:

protamine 1 mg/1 mg heparin

☞ *Administer slowly to avoid severe hypotension and pulmonary HTN.*

☞ *Beware of potential anaphylactic reactions in patients on NPH, with prior exposure to protamine or with fish allergy.*

CAUSES OF HYPOTENSION PROBLEMS

HYPOTENSION (MAP <40 mm Hg) DURING BYPASS

Remember MAP = CO (pump flow rate) × SVR (phenylephrine)

Preload deficit:
> hypovolemia, bleeding, venous cannula malfunction

Afterload deficit:
> vasodilation, aortic dissection, arterial cannula malfunction

Contractility deficit:
> low pump flow

LOW CO PROBLEMS COMING OFF BYPASS

ANATOMIC APPROACH

Blood:
> hypovolemia, bleeding, air embolism, coagulopathy

Graft:
> kink, air lock, thrombus

Coronary artery:
> spasm

LV:
> MI, arrhythmias, CHF, tamponade

Ambient factors:
> hypothermia, hypocalcemia, hyperkalemia, acidosis

PHYSIOLOGIC APPROACH				
	Preload **PCWP**	Afterload **SVR**	Contractility **CO**	TREATMENT
Preload problem: hypovolemia...	low	high	low	IV fluid
Afterload problem vasodilation, shock...	low	low	high	vasoconstrictors
Contractility problem MI, CHF...	high	high	low	inotropes, IABP*

Intra-Aortic Balloon Pump (IABP):
> *Balloon inflates during diastole to increase coronary blood flow.*
> *Balloon deflates during systole to decrease afterload.*
> *(Contraindicated in the presence of AR or aortic aneurysm .)*

HYPOTENSION AFTER BYPASS

Preload deficit:

bleeding from platelet dysfunction, inadequate surgical hemostasis, inadequate heparin reversal, protamine anticoagulation, DIC

cardiac *tamponade*

Afterload deficit:

vasodilation from rewarming

Contractility deficit:

MI, low cardiac output syndrome, graft kink

acidosis, hypothermia

16

VASCULAR SURGERY

The main cause of perioperative mortality & morbidity is **cardiac**.

ABDOMINAL AORTIC ANEURYSM (AAA)

Size over 5 cm is considered for surgery.
  5% mortality for elective surgery.
50% mortality for emergency surgery.

The goal is to prevent MI and acute renal failure (ARF):
  CAD from atherosclerosis, HTN, smoking is prevalent (70%) in the patient population.
  Infrarenal clamping can still cause renal failure.

MANAGEMENT
PRE-OP
  Evaluate for end-organ dysfunctions:
    Heart: Establish baseline hemodynamics via PAC in addition to other cardiac tests.
    Kidney: Check BUN/creatinine.
    Lung: Check CXR; consider ABG/PFT.

  Consider epidural anesthesia/analgesia:
    Heparinization after the catheter placement is acceptable.

  Prepare for major blood loss:
    Have a cell saver and adequate blood products available.
    Establish adequate IV access.

INTRA-OP
    Maintain stable hemodynamics during induction, aortic clamping/unclamping:
        Monitor hemodynamics closely via A-line/PAC.
        Anticipate preload/afterload changes with aortic clamping/unclamping.
        Keep up with blood loss.

    Maintain kidney perfusion:
        Monitor urine output closely.
        Administer fluid/diuretics. (Prophylactic administration of diuretics is not recommended.)
        Keep up with blood loss.

POST-OP
    Monitor end-organ functions:
        Rule out MI, ARF, CVA, etc..
        Rule out post-op bleeding.

    Maintain stable hemodynamics:
        Control pain with continuous epidural analgesia.
        Consider post-op ventilatory support.

THORACIC AORTIC ANEURYSM

A right radial A-line is preferred in case of left subclavian artery clamping.
An additional A-line is placed in the lower extremity to monitor the MAP below the aortic clamping.
A double-lumen ETT is useful in case of thoracotomy.
CPB is often required.
Major complications include paraplegia and acute renal failure.

RISK FACTORS
HTN, pregnancy
Marfan syndrome, Ehlers-Danlos syndrome
deceleration injury (tear of ligamentum arteriosum), post cardiac surgery

SIGNS & SYMPTOMS
chest pain, AR, decreased distal pulse, tamponade, mediastinal shadow

MANAGEMENT
PRE-OP
    Maintain adequate hydration:
        Establish adequate IV access.
    Prevent further dissection:
        Keep SBP <100 mm Hg with nitroprusside, esmolol, trimethaphan.
        Keep contractility low.
        Keep HR low.

INTRA-OP
    Preserve brain, heart, spinal cord, and kidney:
        Keep MAP >100 mm Hg <u>above</u> the aortic clamping.
        Keep MAP > 50 mm Hg <u>below</u> the aortic clamping.

POST-OP
    Monitor the end-organ functions.

SPINAL CORD BLOOD SUPPLY & PRESERVATION

BLOOD SUPPLY

Spinal cord arteries originate from vertebral artery and aorta.

1 Anterior spinal artery:
   Provides 75% of blood flow to the anterior 2/3 of spinal cord.
   Has poor collateral circulation.
   Supplemented by 3 radicular arteries (cervical, upper thoracic, thoracolumbar).
   The thoracolumbar radicular artery is also known as
   the artery of Adamkowicz, which mainly arises between T9-12 levels.

2 Posterior spinal arteries:
   Provide 25% of blood flow to the posterior 1/3 of spinal cord.
   Have good collateral circulation.

PRESERVATION

Spinal cord perfusion pressure = DBP − CSF pressure.
Consider SSEP to detect spinal ischemia (unreliable).
Keep the clamping time below 30 minutes.
Hypothermia, mannitol, steroid, or CSF drainage may be helpful.

CAROTID ENDARTERECTOMY

ANESTHETIC CONCERNS
The goal is to prevent MI, CVA:
☞ *Evaluate for end-organ dysfunctions.*
MI is the major cause of post-op complication.
CVA usually occurs from thromboembolism, not hypotension.

Check coagulation status as the patients are often on aspirin or Coumadin.
Check for carotid obstruction with the head position changes.

INDICATIONS
Transient ischemic attack (TIA):
A temporary (<24 h) neurological deficit from thromboembolism of sclerotic plaque.
A major CVA occurs in 30% within 5 years.
Severe stenosis (>70% occlusion) :
A bruit may not be heard in case of severe stenosis.
Ulcerated plaques

GA vs. CERVICAL PLEXUS BLOCK (C2-4)
Mortality & morbidity are similar.
The regional technique allows mental status monitoring,
 but hemodynamic changes may be more pronounced in an awake patient.
Deep GA with phenylephrine to maintain BP increases the risk for MI.

CBF MAINTENANCE & MONITORING
MAP:
Maintain at a high to normal level to adequately perfuse the brain.
PCO$_2$:
Maintain normocarbia to avoid cerebral vasoconstriction.
Shunt:
Thromboembolism may occur during the placement.
Stump pressure:
Reflects collateral circulatory pressure through the circle of Willis (Figure 2).
Maintain above 60 mm Hg (unreliable).
SSEP:
Does not monitor motor pathways.
EEG:
Reflects global function, not focal function (reliable).

POST-OP COMPLICATIONS

CNS
    CVA:
    usually occurs from thromboembolism, not hypotension

LUNG
    Airway obstruction:
    from hematoma, recurrent laryngeal nerve injury, cranial nerve injury
    Hypoventilation:
    from carotid body injury (decreased ventilatory drive to low PO_2)

HEART
    MI:
    major cause of perioperative mortality/ morbidity
    Hemodynamic instability:
    from carotid sinus injury

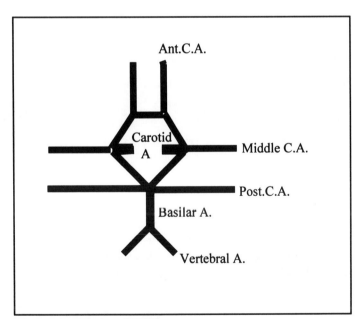

Figure 2. Circle of Willis

17

EYE SURGERY

Mydriasis is "large." (sympathetic pupillary dilation)
Miosis is "small." (parasympathetic pupillary constriction)

INTRAOCULAR PRESSURE (IOP)

IOP is increased by:
ABC problems:
   hypoxemia, **hypercarbia**, hypertension

Aqueous **humor** congestion:
   glaucoma

Blood congestion:
   increased CVP from cough, bucking

Periocular **muscle** contraction:
   succinylcholine, ketamine

Intraocular **gas** expansion:
   $SF_6 + N_2O$

Anesthetic agents in general decrease IOP *except*:
Succinylcholine:
   Increases IOP by 5-10 mm Hg for 5-10 minutes.
   Never been implicated for actual extrusion of the eye content in open eye injury
   when pretreated with a nondepolarizing muscle relaxant (*controversial*).

Ketamine:
   Causes blepharospasm and nystagmus.

N_2O:
   Expands the intraocular gas bubbles.

OCULOCARDIAC REFLEX

Complications:
    Bradyarrhythmias, hypotension, or asystole

Pathophysiology:
    Usually caused by surgical traction of the extraocular muscles.
    The neural pathway consists of trigeminal nerve (5) to vagus (10).
    Aggravated by **hypoxemia**, **hypercarbia** and light anesthesia.
    Prevented by anticholinergics IV (not IM) and retrobulbar block.

Management:
    Treatment includes removal of the stimulus, deepening of the anesthesia,
    anticholinergics and local anesthetic infiltration of the extraocular muscles.

RETROBULBAR BLOCK

Contraindications:
    coagulopathy
    open eye injury

Complications:
    eye injection   (oculocardiac reflex, global perforation, optic nerve injury)
    vascular injection   (bleeding/hematoma, seizures)
    intrathecal injection (delayed apnea)

OPEN EYE INJURY

Administer Bicitra, Reglan, H_2 blockers.
Ascertain that muscle relaxation is complete before attempting direct laryngoscopy:
☞ *Use a muscle twitch monitor.*
Succinylcholine has never been implicated for extrusion of the eye content
when pretreated with a non-depolarizing muscle relaxant (*controversial*).
☞ *Do not lose the airway to save an eye.*

STRABISMUS

Succinylcholine interferes with the forced duction test for 20 minutes.
There is an increased incidence of MH among the patient population.
There is an increased incidence of nausea/vomiting post-op.

CORNEAL ABRASION

The patient complains of "sandy," teary, and painful eyes.
It usually resolves within 2 days.
Treatment includes application of antibiotic ointment.

DRUG INTERACTIONS

Anesthetic	Ophthalmic	Action	Complication	Prevention
N_2O	SF_6	used to treat retina detachment	air bubble expansion	Avoid N_2O 15 min before & for 1 month after SF_6.
succinylcholine	echothiophate	irreversibly inhibits pseudo-cholinesterases	prolonged muscle relaxation	Monitor the muscle twitch response. Stop echothiophate 1 month before OR.

18

CNS PROBLEMS

NEUROPSYCHIATRIC ILLNESSES

DEPRESSION
Consider the drug effects on patients.
Consider the drug effects on anesthetics.

TRICYCLIC ANTIDEPRESSANTS
nortriptyline (Pamelor), amitriptyline (Elavil), imipramine (Tofranil), doxepin (Sinequan)

Action:
Increase postsynaptic [NE] by blocking the <u>uptake</u>.
anticholinergic effects, sedation, arrhythmias

Side effects:
Decrease MAC.
HTN, arrhythmias may occur with sympathetic activation:
☞ *Avoid halothane, pancuronium, ketamine, ephedrine, or epinephrine in the local anesthetics.*

MONOAMINE OXIDASE (MAO) INHIBITORS
phenelzine(Nardil), isocarboxazid(Marplan), tranylcypromine(Parnate), pargyline(Eutonyl)

Action:
Increase postsynaptic [NE] by blocking the <u>breakdown</u>.

Side effects:
Increase MAC.
Hypertensive crisis may occur with tyramine in cheese, wine, ephedrine.
☞ *Neuroleptic malignant hyperthermia may occur with Demerol or other opioids.*

LITHIUM

☞ *Stop lithium 2 weeks before OR.*

Side effects of lithium:
  Decreases MAC.
  seizures
  arrhythmias, hypotension
  muscle weakness, hypothyroidism, DI

ELECTROCONVULSIVE THERAPY (ECT)

Contraindications:
  increased ICP
  recent MI (<3 months) or CVA (<1 month)
  cerebral or aortic aneurysms, pheochromocytoma, pregnancy

Complications:
  bradytachyarrhythmias

SCHIZOPHRENIA

Pathophysiology:
  increased dopaminergic neurotransmission

Anesthetic concerns:
  Anti-psychotic drugs are antidopaminergic.
  Anti-psychotic drugs cause orthostatic hypotension from alpha blockade.

Neuroleptic malignant hyperthermia:
  May occur with anti-dopaminergic drugs including droperidol or Reglan
  that affect the thermoregulatory center in the hypothalamus.
  Treatment includes bromocriptine (a dopamine agonist) and dantrolene.

PARKINSON'S DISEASE

Pathophysiology:
  dopamine (DA) deficiency in basal ganglia
  ☞ *Avoid anti-dopaminergic drugs (droperidol, Reglan).*

Anesthetic concerns:
  Levodopa increases [DA], causing hypertension, tachycardia, hypovolemia, N/V.

DOWN SYNDROME (TRISOMY 21)

Pathophysiology:
   a chromosome defect

Anesthetic concern:
   atlas-axis instability
☞ *Check the C-spine.*
   difficult airway? (subglottic stenosis, large tongue)
   pulmonary HTN/congenital heart diseases
   seizures

CEREBRAL PALSY (CP)

Pathophysiology:
   a hypoxic cerebral injury

Anesthetic concerns:
   muscle contractures (problematic for positioning, ventilation)
   Succinylcholine does not cause massive hyperkalemia.
   respiratory failure/aspiration (kyphoscoliosis/gastroesophageal reflux)
   seizures
   hypothermia

MULTIPLE SCLEROSIS (MS)

Pathophysiology:
   demyelination of CNS

Anesthetic concerns:
   abnormal airway reflex/aspiration
   hemodynamic instability from autonomic nervous system dysfunction
☞ *Heat/fever, spinal anesthesia aggravate the disease.*
☞ *Avoid succinylcholine.*

AMYOTROPHIC LATERAL SCLEROSIS (ALS)

Pathophysiology:
   degeneration of CNS motor neurons

Anesthetic concerns:
   respiratory failure/aspiration
☞ *Avoid succinylcholine.*

GUILLAIN-BARRÉ SYNDROME

Pathophysiology:
   demyelination of CNS including autonomic nervous system

Anesthetic concerns:
   respiratory failure/aspiration
   hemodynamic instability from autonomic nervous system dysfunction
☞ *Avoid succinylcholine.*

MYELOMENINGOCELE (SPINA BIFIDA)

Pathophysiology:
   lack of skin covering for a neural sac

Anesthetic concerns:
   latex allergy
   VATER syndrome
   Succinylcholine does not cause massive hyperkalemia.
   Arnold-Chiari malformation (hindbrain displacement)
   hydrocephalus
   seizures
   respiratory failure/aspiration (from kyphoscoliosis/abnormal airway reflex)
   positioning

ELDERLY PATIENTS

☞ Rule out sepsis, dehydration, drug toxicity.
☞ Rule out CVA, arrhythmias, and other cardiac problems

AGING & PHYSIOLOGIC CHANGES
All organ systems are involved.

CNS
MAC, airway reflex, local anesthetic requirement for regional anesthesia decrease.

HEART
Beta-adrenergic receptor sensitivity, CO, conduction, vascular compliance decrease.
(systolic HTN, LVH, bradycardia)

LUNG
PaO_2 (= 100 – [age/3]), VC, chest wall compliance decrease.
FRC, CC, dead space increase.
(kyphoscoliosis)

KIDNEY
GFR, clearance decrease.
Volume of distribution (for the lipid-soluble), elimination half-life increase.

LIVER
Hepatic blood flow, [albumin] decrease.

GI
Gastric emptying slows down.

ENDOCRINE
DM, hypothyroidism occur more often.

MUSCULOSKELETAL
Fat tissue content increases.
Arthritis, osteoporosis, skin atrophy are common.

ALZHEIMER'S DISEASE

Avoid anticholinergics as patient's acetylcholine is depleted in brain.
Avoid sedatives.

SUBSTANCE ABUSE

ALCOHOLISM
MAC is decreased in acute intoxication.
MAC is increased in chronic abuse.

EFFECTS ON ORGAN SYSTEMS
CNS
encephalopathy, neuropathy
hypoglycemia
seizures from withdrawal (D&T)

HEART
dilated cardiomyopathy
cardiac depression

LUNG
respiratory depression
aspiration, pneumonia
bronchitis from concurrent smoking

GI/LIVER
full stomach
cirrhosis, esophageal varices
acute hepatitis, acute pancreatitis

KIDNEY
diuresis from decreased ADH response

BLOOD
anemia, thrombocytopenia

COCAINE

Inhibits the NE uptake; directly acts on DA receptors.
Metabolized by plasma cholinesterase.
During acute intoxication, massive sympathetic activation can lead to
MI, arrhythmias, CVA , seizures, hyperthermia.
Beware of unopposed alpha stimulation when using beta blockers.
Chronic abuse can result in cardiomyopathy.

19

REGIONAL ANESTHESIA

LEVEL OF INNERVATION

C3-5:	diaphragm
C5-T1:	arm (brachial plexus)
T1-4:	cardiac accelerating fibers
T4:	nipple, carina
T6:	xiphoid process, the lowest point of thoracic curvature
T10:	umbilicus, bladder
L1:	inguinal ligament

SPINAL & EPIDURAL ANESTHESIA

CONTRAINDICATIONS

ABSOLUTE

patient refusal
coagulopathy
infection at the injection site
hypovolemia

RELATIVE

no patient cooperation
anti-platelet drugs (e.g., ASA)
sepsis/bacteremia
chronic progressive neurological diseases (e.g., multiple sclerosis)
chronic back pain/previous back surgery
AS, IHSS, R to L shunt
increased ICP

COMPLICATIONS
Always occur during the examination.

COMMON
Hypotension:
    from decreased venous return from venodilation
    from decreased HR if cardiac accelerating fibers (T1-4) are blocked

Nausea/vomiting:
    from hypotension causing medullary brainstem ischemia
    from unopposed vagal stimulation

Dural puncture headache:
    more likely if young, female, pregnant
    more likely if the needle is large
    worse when sitting-up; occipital/frontal
    The ultimate treatment is blood patch (10-20 ml; 94% success rate).

RARE
High spinal :
    " whispering," " weak upper extremities"

    blockade above T4 (above T6 in COPD)
    respiratory failure:
        from hypotension causing respiratory center ischemia
        from paralysis of diaphragm (C3-5 block)
        from paralysis of intercostals in COPD
    bradycardia/hypotension

Intravascular injection (epidural):
    "ringing in the ear," "metallic taste"

    <u>CNS</u>   toxicity causing seizures
    <u>cardiac</u> toxicity causing cardiac arrest

EXTREMELY RARE
Neurological injury:
    <u>physical</u> nerve injury (needle, catheter, hematoma)
    <u>chemical</u> nerve injury (chloroprocaine)

Infection:
    meningitis
    abscess

COMPARISON OF SPINAL & EPIDURAL ANESTHESIA

ADVANTAGES
SPINAL & EPIDURAL ANESTHESIA OVER GENERAL ANESTHESIA

Both avoid airway instrumentation
Both block adrenal response to surgery.
Both reduce blood loss & incidence of DVT in lower extremity surgeries.
Both allow monitoring for mental status changes, chest pain or positional injuries.

SPINAL ANESTHESIA

Provides a reliable, dense block.
Quick, easy to perform.
Requires very little local anesthetics (no toxicity).

EPIDURAL ANESTHESIA

Provides more control with onset, level and duration of the block.
Avoids potential dural puncture headache when performed correctly.
May be used for post-op analgesia.

FACTORS INFLUENCING THE EXTENT OF BLOCKADE
SPINAL ANESTHESIA

Patient:
   age, height
   intra-abdominal pressure (pregnancy, ascites, obesity)
   position
Local anesthetic:
   dosage, volume
   baricity (= density of the local anesthetic/density of CSF)
   speed of injection

EPIDURAL ANESTHESIA

Patient:
   age, height
   intra-abdominal pressure (pregnancy, ascites, obesity)
   site of injection
Local anesthetic:
   dosage, volume

UPPER EXTREMITY BLOCKS

INNERVATION OF THE UPPER EXTREMITY

BRACHIAL PLEXUS (C5-T1) (Figure 3)
Musculocutaneous nerve (MC):
> Early branching through coracobrachialis may require direct injection into the muscle.

Median nerve (M):
> located medial to brachial artery

Radial nerve (R):
> located posterior to axillary artery

Ulnar nerve (U):
> located between olecranon and medial epicondyle

Cutaneous nerves:
> medial brachial cutaneous nerve (C8-T1)
> intercostobrachial nerve (T2)

AXILLARY BLOCK

Good for the distal half of the upper extremity (ulnar distribution).
May miss musculocutaneous nerve due to early branching through coracobrachialis.

Landmarks:
> axillary artery, pectoralis major

INTERSCALENE BLOCK

Good for the proximal half of the upper extremity including shoulder.
May miss ulnar nerve due to the lowest position within brachial plexus.

Landmarks:
> cricoid cartilage, sternocleidomastoid, anterior & middle scalene

Complications:

vertebral artery injection	(seizures, cardiac arrest)
intrathecal/epidural injection	(total spinal)
stellate ganglion block	(Horner's sign)
phrenic nerve block	(respiratory failure from hemi-diaphragm paresis)
recurrent laryngeal nerve block	(hoarseness)
lung puncture	(pneumothorax)

Rapid-Sequence Review of Anesthesiology

BIER BLOCK

Use 50 ml of lidocaine 0.5% **without epinephrine**.

Check the tourniquet; keep the pressure 100 mm Hg above the SBP.

☞ *Do not deflate the tourniquet if lidocaine was injected less than 30 minutes ago.*

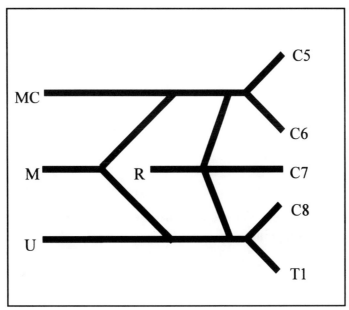

Figure 3. Brachial plexus

LOWER EXTREMITY BLOCKS

INNERVATION OF THE LOWER EXTREMITY

LUMBAR PLEXUS (L1-4)
Femoral nerve (L2-4):
saphenous nerve (subcutaneous)

Lateral femoral cutaneous nerve (L1-3)
Obturator nerve (L2-4)

SACRAL PLEXUS (L4-S2)
Sciatic nerve (L4-S2)
Tibial nerve:
posterior tibial nerve
sural nerve (subcutaneous)

Peroneal nerve:
deep peroneal nerve
superficial peroneal nerve (subcutaneous)

ANKLE BLOCK

5 nerves to be blocked: 2 deep, 3 subcutaneous (see the **bolds** above).
Contraindicated if the foot is infected.

LOCAL ANESTHETICS

PHARMACODYNAMICS
Block Na^+ channel.

PHARMACOKINETICS
Potency is proportional to <u>lipid solubility.</u>
Onset is proportional to <u>the fraction of non-ionized portion (pK).</u>
Duration is proportional to <u>protein binding.</u>

SIGNS & SYMPTOMS OF SYSTEMIC TOXICITY
Aggravated by **hypoxemia**, **hypercarbia**, acidosis, pregnancy

CNS:
   metallic taste, ringing in the ear, slurred speech
   confusion, excitation
   seizures, loss of consciousness, apnea

Heart:
   hypotension, arrhythmias
   asystole

TYPES OF LOCAL ANESTHETICS
Esters:
   procaine, chloroprocaine, tetracaine, cocaine *(one 'I' in the generic name)*
   metabolized by pseudocholinesterase
   A metabolite, PABA, can cause allergic reaction.

Amides:
   all others including lidocaine, bupivacaine   *(two 'I's in the generic name)*
   metabolized by liver
   The preservative, methylparaben, can cause allergic reaction.

COMMON LOCAL ANESTHETICS

Name	Maximum Dose	Duration **	Usage	Comments
procaine (Novocaine)	12 mg/kg	0.5-1 h	spinal epidural infiltration	
chloroprocaine (Nesacaine)	12 mg/kg	0.5-1 h	epidural infiltration	☞Do not use for spinal: low pH & bisulfite preservative may cause neurological injuries
cocaine	3 mg/kg	0.5-2 h	topical	sympathetic activation
tetracaine (Pontocaine)	3 mg/kg	2-3 h 3-5 h with epi	topical spinal	provides good motor block
lidocaine (Xylocaine)	5 mg/kg 7 mg/kg with epi	1-1.5 h	topical spinal epidural infiltration	an antiarrhythmic suppresses airway reflex causes CNS sedation/seizure potentiates inhalational agents
bupivacaine (Marcaine, Sensorcaine)	3 mg/kg	2-4 h	spinal epidural infiltration	☞Do not use 0.75% solution for epidural in pregnant patients: unresponsive to resuscitation in case of cardiotoxicity

* Maximum dose increases with the addition of epinephrine by 25-50% in approximation.

**Duration increases with the addition of epinephrine by 50-100% in approximation.

☞Never add epinephrine to the local anesthetics when using for digital, penile, or Bier block.

20
PAIN

Causalgia:
> sympathetic nervous system dysfunction from a major *nerve trunk* injury

Allodynia:
> pain from non-painful stimuli

Hyperesthesia:
> increased sensitivity to touch

REFLEX SYMPATHETIC DYSTROPHY (RSD)

DEFINITION
A pain syndrome that occurs
(*History*) after major or minor trauma to bone or soft tissue,
(*Pain*) characterized by burning, aching pain disproportionate to the injury, and
(*Autonomic nervous system*) vasomotor changes and atrophy, which is responsive to sympathetic denervation.

PATHOPHYSIOLOGY
Abnormal synapses form between sympathetic and somatic neural pathways after demyelination from the trauma.

SIGNS & SYMPTOMS
Pain:
> burning, aching, not consistent with dermatomal distribution

Vasomotor changes:
> cold, clammy, cyanotic extremities

Atrophy:
> hair loss, nail changes, skin changes, muscle and bone wasting

TREATMENT

Sympathectomy:
    chemical (local anesthetics, alcohol)
    surgical

IV regional block:
    reserpine, guanethidine, bretylium
    depletes NE at nerve endings and changes pain receptor sensitivity

Systemic medications:
    alpha, beta blockers; steroids

Physical therapy

SYMPATHETIC GANGLION BLOCKS

STELLATE GANGLION BLOCK (C7)

Horner's sign:
ptosis, miosis, anhidrosis caused by stellate ganglion block

Indications:
upper extremity with vascular insufficiency or RSD

Landmarks:
Chassaignac's tubercle (C6 transverse process), cricoid cartilage (C6)

Complications:

vertebral artery injection	(seizures, cardiac arrest)
intrathecal/epidural injection	(total spinal)
phrenic nerve block	(hemiparesis of diaphragm)
recurrent laryngeal nerve block	("lump", hoarseness)
brachial plexus block	(arm weakness)
lung puncture	(pneumothorax)
neck hematoma	(airway obstruction)

LUMBAR SYMPATHETIC BLOCK (L2)

Indications:
lower extremity with vascular insufficiency or RSD

Landmarks:
L2

Complications:

genitofemoral nerve injury	(groin pain)
kidney/ureter injury	(hematuria)
vascular injection	(seizures, cardiac arrest)
intrathecal/epidural injection	(total spinal)
lumbar disc injury	(back pain)

CELIAC PLEXUS BLOCK (L1)

Indications:
    pancreatic cancer pain

Landmarks:
    L1

Complications:

sympathetic block	(hypotension, diarrhea from increased peristalsis)
diaphragmatic irritation	(shoulder pain)
vascular injection	(seizures, cardiac arrest)
intrathecal/epidural injection	(total spinal)
lumbar disc	(back pain)

21

MACHINES & PHYSICS

Is the patient's problem from the patient or the machine?

ELECTRICITY

Macroshock occurs at *100 mA* through skin to heart.
Micro shock occurs at *100 μA* through direct contact to heart via an intracardiac wire.
The maximum current leakage should be under *10 μA* for OR equipment.

LINE ISOLATION MONITOR

Alarms when potential current flow from the power source to ground exceeds 5 mA.
Does not protect from microshock.

☞ *Unplug each piece of equipment to identify the source of current leakage.*

ELECTROCAUTERY ("Bovie")

Uses a high frequency to minimize triggering VF.
The current travels through the body.
Heat is generated from the high current density.

☞ *The dispersive pad should be applied to skin evenly to avoid a burn injury.*

LASER

LIGHT AMPLIFICATION OF THE STIMULATED EMISSION OF RADIATION

Provides precision and coagulation.
Minimizes edema and scarring.

GASES
CO_2:
  superficial penetration
  good for precise work on all tissues
  causes minimal tissue edema

Neodymium-doped yttrium-aluminum-garnet (Nd:YAG):
  deep penetration
  good for coagulation work on darkly pigmented tissue
  can cause ignition

PRECAUTIONS
Beware of **airway fire**:
  Use a proper ETT to avoid ignition (a foil-wrapped red rubber tube/a stainless-steel tube).
  Fill the cuff with NS or an inert dye solution (to help detecting perforation).
  Use air or helium with the lowest FIO_2. (N_2O supports combustion.)

Beware of **eye injury**:
  Protect eyes by covering both yours and the patient's.

Beware of post-op **airway edema**:
  Consider steroids.

AIRWAY FIRE
Disconnect the ventilatory circuit from the ETT.
Remove the ETT.
Flush the area with NS.
Replace the ETT, and ventilate with 100% O_2.
Perform bronchoscopy/lavage.
Monitor in ICU for ventilatory support.

VENTILATOR/CIRCUITS

VENTILATORY MODES IN ICU

CONTROLLED MANDATORY VENTILATION (CMV)
Only the ventilator does all the breathing.

INTERMITTENT MANDATORY VENTILATION (IMV)
The ventilator does the breathing; the patient can also breathe spontaneously.
This mode lowers the mean airway pressure; useful for weaning.

SYNCHRONIZED INTERMITTENT MANDATORY VENTILATION (SIMV)
IMV in which the patient's spontaneous breathing is synchronized
to the mechanical ventilation.

ASSISTED-CONTROLLED VENTILATION (ACV)
The ventilator delivers the preset tidal volume when the patient attempts to breathe.

PRESSURE SUPPORT VENTILATION (PSV)
The ventilator gives "a little push" when the patient attempts to breathe.

POSITIVE END-EXPIRATORY PRESSURE (PEEP)
The ventilator keeps the patient's lung inflated throughout the mechanical ventilation cycle.
Indicated for PaO_2 <60 mm Hg on FIO_2 >60%.
Increases FRC; decreases shunting.
Decreases venous return and CO.
May cause pneumothorax.

CONTINUOUS POSITIVE AIRWAY PRESSURE (CPAP)
The ventilator keeps the patient's lung inflated while he is breathing spontaneously.
Aspiration may occur if the airway reflex is not adequate.

MAPLESON CIRCUITS

Circuit components:
   a fresh gas inlet, a corrugated tube, a reservoir bag, an expiratory valve

ADVANTAGES

Lower resistance/work of breathing during spontaneous ventilation
as unidirectional valves and a CO_2 absorber are absent.
light, portable

DISADVANTAGES

Require high fresh gas flow to avoid CO_2 rebreathing.

VARIATIONS (A through F)

Bain circuit (D):
   Coaxial arrangement warms the inspiratory gas with expiratory flow.
   Kinks and disconnection may occur without notice.

Ayre's-T piece (E):
   useful for weaning an intubated patient from a ventilator.

Jackson-Rees modification (F):
   popular for pediatric patients

Order of preference:
   spontaneous ventilation (ADCB)
   controlled   ventilation (DBCA)

RELATIVE POSITION OF THE CIRCUIT COMPONENTS TO THE PATIENT

CIRCUIT	0	1	2	3	4
Mapleson A	Patient	Valve	Tube	Bag	Gas inlet
Mapleson B	Patient	Valve	Gas inlet	Tube	Bag
Mapleson C	Patient	Valve	Gas inlet	Bag	
Mapleson D	Patient	Gas inlet	Tube	Valve	Bag
Mapleson E	Patient	Gas inlet	Tube		
Mapleson F	Patient	Gas inlet	Tube	Bag	Valve

MONITORS

"What are the ASA standard monitors (8)?"

Oxygenation: a pulse oximeter, an oxygen analyzer
Ventilation: a capnography, a precordial stethoscope, a disconnection alarm
Circulation: a BP cuff, ECG
Temperature: a temperature probe

PULSE OXIMETER

<u>Deoxygenated</u> Hb absorbs light at <u>660</u> nm wavelength (red).
  <u>Oxygenated</u> Hb absorbs light at <u>940</u> nm wavelength (infrared).
SpO_2 can be calculated based on the different absorptions.
Carboxy-Hb is read as SpO_2 of 100%.
    Met-Hb is read as SpO_2 of   85%.

MASS SPECTROMETER

Gas molecules are bombarded by an electron beam and ionized.
The ionized molecules are deflected by a magnetic field
according to the molecular weight/charge ratio.
A collector plate measures the scattered molecules by the molecular weight/charge ratio.
The concentration and the identity of the gas molecules are recognized.

ELECTROENCEPHALOGRAM (EEG)

Monitors global cerebral ischemia from inadequate CBF.
The injury results in low frequency & amplitude.
Hypoxia, hypotension, hypothermia, anesthetics also cause low frequency & amplitude.
Does not detect the injury to a focal area or deep structures.

SOMATOSENSORY EVOKED POTENTIALS (SSEP)

Monitors spinal cord posterior column (sensory pathway) integrity.
The injury results in prolonged latency & decreased amplitude.
Hypoxia, hypotension, hypothermia, anesthetics also cause
prolonged latency & decreased amplitude.
Does not detect the injury to the anterior column (motor pathway).

22

COMMON DRUGS

The drugs in this chapter represent only a part of all the drugs we need to know about. The dosages are only approximations.

*Pharmacodynamics: what the **drug** **d**oes to the body*
Pharmacokinetics: what the body does to the drug

INDUCTION AGENTS

All can induce hypnosis (unconsciousness), apnea, and loss of airway reflex.

Drug	Dose	Action	Side effects	Comments
thiopental (Pentothal)	4-6 mg/kg	rapid redistribution anticonvulsant	histamine release hypotension bronchospasm (?)	can precipitate porphyria in the susceptible
propofol (Diprivan)	2-2.5mg/kg	rapid metabolism without accumulation clear recovery	hypotension by low SVR pain with injection	Beware of bacteremia. (Use within 6 h)
etomidate	0.3 mg/kg	stable hemodynamics	nausea/vomiting adrenal suppression activates seizure foci/myoclonus	recommended for critically ill, cardiac patients
ketamine	1-2 mg/kg	sympathetic activation bronchodilation analgesia	nightmare/delirium profuse secretion increased ICP/IOP	Administer with benzodiazepine, anticholinergics
methohexital (Brevital)	1-2 mg/kg	short duration	seizure foci activation	popular for ECT & cardioversion

INHALATIONAL AGENTS

MAC

MAC reflects <u>potency</u>.

Definition:

Minimum Alveolar Concentration at which 50% of the patients do not respond to the surgical incision.

MAC is **increased** by:

hyperthermia, hypernatremia
chronic alcohol abuse; acute amphetamine/cocaine use
MAO inhibitors, tricyclic antidepressants

MAC is **decreased** by:

hypothermia, hyponatremia
acute alcohol intoxication; chronic amphetamine abuse
methyldopa, clonidine, lithium, anesthetics
PaO_2 <40 mm Hg, $PaCO_2$ >95 mm Hg, MAP <40 mm Hg, Hct <10%
pregnancy, extreme age (premies, geriatrics)

RATE (SPEED) OF INDUCTION

Input:

inspired partial pressure* (FI)
breathing system
alveolar ventilation (FRC, MV)

Uptake:

alveolar-venous partial pressure gradient
solubility**
CO

* partial pressure – concentration of gas – gas tension
**solubility = blood/gas partition coefficient (The higher the solubility; the slower the induction.)

GENERAL EFFECTS ON ORGAN SYSTEMS
CNS
  Increase CBF/ICP.
  Decrease $CMRO_2$.

HEART
  Decrease BP/CO.

LUNG
  Decrease TV/MV; increase RR.
  Decrease the ventilatory drive response to PCO_2.
  Eliminate the ventilatory drive response to PO_2.
  Cause bronchodilation.
  Decrease HPV response only at very high concentrations.

KIDNEY
  Decrease RBF.
  F⁻ nephrotoxicity possible with enflurane.

COMPARISONS OF THE INHALATIONAL AGENTS

Agent	MAC (%)	Blood/Gas P.C.	CV effects	Side effects/Comments
halothane	0.74	2.4	maintains SVR decreases HR decreases contractility	arrhythmias with catecholamines, halothane hepatitis
enflurane	1.7	1.8	decreases SVR decreases contractility	seizures increased CSF production F⁻ nephrotoxicity
isoflurane	1.14	1.4	decreases SVR increases HR maintains CO	coronary steal (?) increased CSF absorption
sevoflurane	2	0.6	decreases contractility	minimal airway irritation F⁻ nephrotoxicity
desflurane	6	0.42	similar to isoflurane	airway irritation
N_2O	104	0.47	increases PVR/SVR decreases CO with LV dysfunction/opioids	gas expansion DNA synthesis inhibition

MUSCLE RELAXANTS

PHASE 1 vs. PHASE 2 BLOCK

	PHASE 1 block	PHASE 2 block
Tetanic fade	no	yes
Post-tetanic potentiation	no	yes
Train-of-four	>70% ratio	<30% ratio
Response to anticholinesterase	prolonged block	reversal
Type of relaxants	depolarizing	nondepolarizing, depolarizing

SUCCINYLCHOLINE

Shelf-life is 14 days.
Made of two acetylcholine molecules.

DEPOLARIZING

Succinylcholine binds to the neuromuscular membrane receptor and precipitates prolonged depolarization, causing it to become unresponsive to subsequent stimuli.

PSEUDOCHOLINESTERASE

(plasma cholinesterase)
hydrolyzes succinylcholine, mivacurium, acetylcholine, trimethaphan and ester local anesthetics (procaine, chloroprocaine, tetracaine, cocaine).
present in plasma
produced by liver
decreased in cirrhosis, pregnancy
inhibited by echothiophate, trimethanphan

Acetylcholinesterase:
Hydrolyzes acetylcholine, physostigmine.
Present in plasma and nerve endings.

RBC esterase:
Hydrolyzes esmolol.

Non-specific (liver) esterase:
Hydrolyzes atracurium.

ATYPICAL PSEUDOCHOLINESTERASE

Atypical pseudocholinesterase cannot hydrolyze succinylcholine in a normal manner due to its qualitative defect and results in prolonged neuromuscular block.
Incidence: 1 in 3,000 (homozygous)

DIBUCAINE

an amide local anesthetics that inhibits pseudocholinesterase:
> normal enzyme: 80% inhibited
> atypical enzyme: 20% inhibited

used to identify atypical pseudocholinesterase.
The result reflects quality, not quantity of pseudocholinesterase.

SIDE EFFECTS OF SUCCINYLCHOLINE

SIDE EFFECTS	RISK FACTORS/COMMENTS
Hyperkalemia/ cardiac arrest	usually 0.5-1 mEq/L increase in $[K^+]$ massive release from proliferation of NMJ in muscular dystrophy, spinal cord injury, burns, crush injury
MH	muscular dystrophy, myotonic dystrophy, osteogenesis imperfecta
Arrhythmias	bradyarrhythmias (especially if second dose is given within 10 min)
Phase 2 block	from prolonged infusion (>2-4 mg/kg)
ICP/IOP/IGP increase	from fasciculations *Precurarization attenuates the increase in ICP.*
Myalgia/ myoglobinuria	from fasciculations young, muscular patients
Prolonged paralysis by decreased pseudocholinesterase activity	qualitative defect: atypical pseudocholinesterase drugs (echothiophate, anticholinesterases) quantitative defect: severe liver disease, pregnancy, hemodialysis
Allergy/anaphylaxis	IgE-mediated

NONDEPOLARIZING MUSCLE RELAXANTS

NONDEPOLARIZING
Binds to the neuromuscular membrane receptors
and competitively inhibits acetylcholine molecules from binding.

TYPES OF NON-DEPOLARIZING MUSCLE RELAXANTS
Steroid:
rocuronium, vecuronium, pancuronium, pipercurium

Benzylisoquinoline:
mivacurium, atracurium, doxacurium

Drug	Intubation Dose	Duration	Primary Route of Elimination	Side effects/Comments
mivacurium	0.2 mg/kg	15-30 min	pseudocholinesterase	histamine release
atracurium	0.5 mg/kg	30-45	Hofmann degradation and ester hydrolysis	histamine release laudanosine: CNS excitation
vecuronium	0.1 mg/kg	30-45	liver	hemodynamic stability
rocuronium	0.6 mg/kg	30-45	liver	precipitation with pentothal rapid onset; CV stability
pancuronium	0.1 mg/kg	60-90	kidney/liver	sympathetic activation
doxacurium	0.05 mg/kg	60-90	kidney	
pipercurium	0.1 mg/kg	60-90	kidney	
tubocurarine	0.5 mg/kg	60-90	kidney	histamine release

FACTORS POTENTIATING MUSCLE RELAXATION
Pharmacologic:
Mg^{++}, lithium, Ca^{++} channel blockers,
inhalational agents,
antibiotics, anticonvulsants, antiarrhythmics (selected ones only)

Metabolic:
hypothermia, hypokalemia,
respiratory acidosis, metabolic alkalosis

REVERSAL AGENTS

Consist of anticholinesterases and anticholinergics.

ANTICHOLINESTERASES

Nicotinic effects:
> Increased [acetylcholine] at NMJ improves skeletal muscle contraction.

Muscarinic effects:
> Increased [acetylcholine] also affects other organ systems causing CNS disturbance, bradycardia, bronchospasm, increased GI motility.

Drug	Dose	Comments
neostigmine	0.035-0.07 mg/kg	more effective than edrophonium for reversing intense neuromuscular blockade
edrophonium	0.5-1 mg/kg	rapid onset: *Administer with atropine rather than glycopyrrolate.*
pyridostigmine	0.1-0.3 mg/kg	delayed onset/longer duration also used for treating myasthenia gravis
physostigmine	0.5-2 mg q15min	crosses BBB/not for reversal antagonizes CNS disturbances caused by scopolamine, atropine, ketamine, benzodiazepines and tricyclics metabolized by acetylcholinesterases

ANTICHOLINERGICS

Antagonize the effect of acetylcholine on muscarinic receptors.

Drug	Dose	Comments
atropine	10-20 µg/kg	best for treating bradycardia
scopolamine	0.4 mg	best for CNS sedation/amnesia minimal tachycardia
glycopyrrolate	10-20 µg/kg for reversal 0.2 mg for drying effect	best for antisialagogue (drying) effect does not cross BBB/no sedation

ANTICHOLINERGIC EFFECTS
CNS
sedation/excitation
mydriasis

HEART
tachycardia

LUNG
decreases airway resistance/increases dead space
drying

GI
decreases GI motility/LES tone

GU
urinary retention

SKIN
decreased sweating/hyperthermia

OPIOIDS

☞ *Naloxone (Narcan) reverses the effects of narcotics, but lasts only 30 minutes.*

Drug	Equivalent Dose	Comments
meperidine (Demerol)	100 mg	tachycardia, hypotension, decreased contractility *Do not administer with MAO inhibitors:* (neuroleptic malignant hyperthermia) stops shivering (12.5-25 mg IV)
morphine	10 mg	histamine release, hypotension, bronchospasm Delayed apnea can occur when given intrathecally.
alfentanil	1 mg	non-accumulative with continuous infusion bradycardia/asystole more likely than with fentanyl
fentanyl	0.1 mg	CV stable
sufentanil	0.01 mg	bradycardia more likely than with fentanyl

EFFECTS OF OPIOIDS

CNS
> miosis
> nausea/vomiting by chemoreceptor trigger zone stimulation
> decrease ICP

HEART
> bradycardia by vagus nuclei stimulation (except Demerol)

LUNG
> depress the ventilatory drive (shifts CO_2 response curve to the right)
> decrease RR/MV, increase TV
> chest wall rigidity interfering with ventilation

GI
> spasm of the Sphincter of Oddi
> constipation, delayed gastric emptying

GU
> urinary retention

PREMEDICATIONS

BENZODIAZEPINES

Potentiate GABA; increase seizure threshold.
Decrease MAC.
Implicated in **birth defects** (cleft palate).
Reversed by flumazenil.

Drug	Dose for Sedation	Half-life	Metabolism	Comments
diazepam (Valium)	10 mg PO (0.2 mg/kg) 2 mg IV (0.05 mg/kg)	24 h	liver	an active metabolite+ painful injection from propylene glycol
midazolam (Versed)	0.5-2 mg IV 0.1 mg/kg IM 0.3 mg/kg intranasally 0.5 mg/kg PO	up to 4 h	liver	

EFFECTS ON ORGAN SYSTEMS
CNS
decrease CBF/ICP
increase seizure threshold

HEART
minimal effect
hypotension, bradycardia in hypovolemic patients

LUNG
decrease the ventilatory drive response to increasing PCO_2

H₂ BLOCKERS

Decrease volume and increase pH of gastric juice secretion.
Do not affect what is already in stomach.
Bronchospasm may occur from the unopposed H$_1$ effect.

Drug	Dose	Comments
ranitidine (Zantac)	150 mg PO 50 mg IV	has fewer side effects than cimetidine
cimetidine (Tagamet)	300 mg PO 300 mg IV	CNS: seizures, confusion Heart: hypotension, arrhythmias Liver: decreased HBF; delayed drug metabolism Blood: gynecomastia, aplastic anemia
famotidine (Pepcid)	20 mg PO 20 mg IV	has fewer side effects than cimetidine can be administered rapidly

ANTIEMETICS

Are antidopaminergic (except ondansetron).
☞ *Do not use in Parkinson's disease.*
Inhibit chemoreceptor trigger zone.
Extrapyramidal symptoms should be treated with benzodiazepines and antihistamines.

Drug	Dose	Comments
metoclopramide (Reglan)	10 mg PO/IV	GI: stimulates gastric emptying; increases LES tone CNS: extrapyramidal symptoms, especially in children Heart: hypertension from catecholamine release *Avoid with MAO inhibitors or in pheochromocytoma.*
droperidol	0.625-2.5 mg IV (15 µg/kg)	CNS: antidopaminergic, neuroleptic Heart: hypotension from alpha$_1$ blockade
ondansetron (Zofran)	4 mg IV	a serotonin antagonist

COMMON DRUGS FOR HEART

SYMPATHETIC NERVOUS SYSTEM

Receptor	End organ	Action	Agonist	Antagonist
Alpha₁	blood vessels bronchioles	constriction	phenylephrine	phentolamine prazosin
Alpha₂	postganglionic sympathetic nerve endings	inhibits NE release (presynaptic)	clonidine	phentolamine
Beta₁	heart	stimulation	dopamine dobutamine isoproterenol	atenolol esmolol propranolol
Beta₂	bronchioles uterus skeletal muscles pulmonary/ coronary vessels	dilation relaxation	albuterol terbutaline isoproterenol	propranolol

VASOPRESSORS/INOTROPES

Drug	Dose	Receptor	Action	Comments
ephedrine	5-10 mg	alpha$_1$ < beta	increases HR, contractility vasoconstriction	indirect > direct acting stimulates NE release. good uterine blood flow tachyphylaxis
phenylephrine (Neosynephrine)	50-100 μg	alpha$_1$	vasoconstriction	reflex bradycardia
dopamine	1-3 μg/kg/min 3-10 10-20	dopa$_1$ beta alpha$_1$	increases RBF increases CO vasoconstriction	*Mix in D5W.*
epinephrine	0.1 μg/kg/min or 1-10 μg/min	alpha$_1$ beta	increases HR, contractility vasoconstriction	arrhythmias
dobutamine (Dobutrex)	2-20μg/kg/min	beta$_1$ >beta$_2$	increases contractility	*Mix in D5W.* For cardiogenic shock
isoproterenol (Isuprel)	0.1 μg/kg/min or 1-10 μg/min	beta	increases HR, contractility decreases SVR/ PVR	For heart blocks
norepinephrine (Levophed)	0.1 μg/kg/min	alpha$_1$ > beta	increases SVR, BP	may decrease HR, CO For septic shock

VASODILATORS/ANTIHYPERTENSIVES

Central sympatholytics:
methyldopa, clonidine

Vasodilators:
hydralazine, nitroglycerin, nitroprusside

Alpha adrenergic blockers:
prazosin, phentolamine

Beta adrenergic blockers:
esmolol, labetolol, propranolol

Calcium channel blockers:
verapamil, nifedipine

Ganglionic blocker:
trimethaphan

Drug	Dose (IV)	Duration	Action	Side effects/Comments
methyldopa (Aldomet)	250-500 mg	12-24 h	alpha$_2$ agonism decreases MAC.	Beta$_2$ blockade can cause HTN. +Coombs test
clonidine (Catapres)	0.2 mg PO,SL,TD 20 µg SPINAL	4-8 h	alpha$_2$ agonism decreases MAC & opioid requirement	rebound HTN if abruptly stopped For opioid withdrawal
hydralazine	5-20 mg	2-4 h	arteriolar smooth muscle relaxation	reflex tachycardia lupus
nitroglycerin	1-10 µg/kg/min	10 min	venodilation: decreases preload & PVR/SVR	increases CBF/ICP reflex tachycardia methemoglobinemia
nitroprusside	1-10 µg/kg/min	10 min	arteria > venous smooth muscle relaxation: decreases SVR	increases CBF/ICP reflex tachycardia CN$^-$ toxicity: tachyphylaxis, acidosis
prazosin	1-2 mg PO	4-6 h	alpha$_1$ blockade	no reflex tachycardia

Drug	Dose (IV)	Duration	Action	Side effects/Comments
phentolamine	2.5-5 mg	10 min	alpha blockade	potentiates beta$_2$ blockade reflex tachycardia
esmolol (Brevibloc)	0.5 mg/kg (loading dose) 0.05 mg/kg/min	10 min	beta$_1$ blockade: decreases HR, contractility	hydrolyzed by RBC esterase
labetalol	5-20 mg	2-4 h	beta >>alpha$_1$ blockade: decreases HR, CO	
propranolol (Inderal)	1-2 mg	1-6 h	beta blockade: decreases HR, contractility	bronchospasm heart blocks, CHF hypoglycemia
verapamil (Calan)	2.5-5 mg	0.5-1 h	slows AV node lowers SVR, CO	used to treat HTN, SVT/AF
nifedipine (Procardia)	10 mg SL	2-4 h	coronary & arterial vasodilation	reflex tachycardia
trimethaphan	10-20 µg/kg/min	10 min	nicotinic ganglion blockade: decreases SVR, CO	eliminated by pseudocholinesterase minimal increase in CBF/ICP mydriasis/cycloplegia tachyphylaxis used in preeclampsia, aortic aneurysms, & cerebral aneurysms

DRUGS MISCELLANEOUS

DRUGS WITH SIMILAR NAMES

AMILORIDE:	a K$^+$-sparing diuretic
AMIODARONE:	an antiarrhythmic for SVT, VT
AMRINONE:	a phosphodiesterase inhibitor used to treat CHF
TRIAMTERENE:	a K$^+$-sparing diuretic
TRIMETHAPHAN:	a ganglionic blocker
PITOCIN (Oxytocin):	a hormone that causes uterine contraction
PITRESSIN (Vasopressin):	an ADH analogue used to treat DI/GI bleeding

DRUGS YOU SHOULD NEVER PUSH IV

Vancomycin:
an antibiotic
Severe hypotension can occur.

Phenytoin (Dilantin):
an anticonvulsant/antiarrhythmic
Heart block/asystole can occur.

Protamine:
a heparin antagonist
Severe hypotension and anaphylaxis can occur.

Aminophylline:
a phosphodiesterase inhibitor used to treat bronchospasm
Arrhythmias and seizures can occur.

Potassium:
an electrolyte
Asystole can occur.

Methylergonovine (Methergine):
an ergot alkaloid used to treat uterine atony and bleeding
Severe hypertension can occur.

DYES & BONE CEMENT

Methylene blue:
is used to treat methemoglobinemia.
can cause hypertension, tachycardia;
incorrect low reading on the pulse oximeter.

Indigo carmine:
can cause hypertension from alpha agonism;
incorrect low reading on the pulse oximeter.

Polymethylmethacrylate:
can cause hypotension and fat embolism.

NEW DRUGS

Cisatracurium (Nimbex):
an isomer of atracurium
eliminated by Hofmann degradation
Unlike atracurium histamine release does not occur.

Remifentanil (Ultiva):
an ultrashort-acting opioid half as potent as fentanyl
eliminated by nonspecific esterase so rapidly that
no residual effect remains within 5 minutes after the infusion is stopped.

Ropivacaine (Naropin):
an amide local anesthetic similar to bupivacaine in duration and potency
less cardiotoxic than bupivacaine
less motor blockade than bupivacaine

References

Barash, PG, Cullen BF, Stoelting RK: *Clinical Anesthesia*, Philadelphia, J. B. Lippincott Company, 1989.

Barash, PG, Cullen BF, Stoelting RK: *Handbook of Clinical Anesthesia*, Philadelphia, J. B. Lippincott Company, 1991.

Braunwald, E et al.: *Harrison's Principles of Internal Medicine: Companion Handbook*, 11th ed., New York, McGraw-Hill, Inc., 1988.

Donegan, JH: *Manual of Anesthesia for Emergency Surgery*, New York, Churchill Livingstone Inc., 1987.

Ehrenwerth, J, Eisenkraft JB: *Anesthesia Equipment: Principles and Applications*, St. Louis, MO, Mosby-Year Book, Inc., 1993.

Ezekiel, MR: *Current Clinical Strategies: Handbook of Anesthesiology*, Fountain Valley, CA, Current Clinical Strategies Publishing, 1995.

Faust RJ: *Anesthesiology Review*, 1st ed., New York, Churchill Livingstone Inc., 1991.

Finucane, BT, Santora, AH: *Principles of Airway Management*, Philadelphia, F. A. Davis Company, 1988.

Firestone, LL, Lebowitz, PW, Cook, CE: *Clinical Anesthesia Procedures of the Massachusetts General Hospital*, 3rd ed., Boston, Little, Brown and Company, 1988.

Gaba, DM, Fish KJ, Howard SK: *Crisis Management in Anesthesiology*, New York, Churchill Livingston Inc., 1994.

Gallagher, CJ, Lubarsky, DA: *Preparing for the Anesthesia Orals: Board Stiff*, Stoneham, MA, Butterworth-Heinemann, 1990.

Gomella, LG et al.: *Clinician's Poket Reference*, 5th ed., Norwalk, CT, Appleton-Century-Crofts, 1986.

Gravenstein, N: *Manual of Complications During Anesthesia*, Philadelphia, J. B. Lippincott Company, 1991.

Jensen, NF: *Anesthesiology Oral Board Prep: The Best Medicine for Your Oral Boards*, Iowa City, IA, 1995.

Marini, JJ, Wheeler, AP: *Critical Care Medicine: The Essentials*, Baltimore, MD, Williams & Wilkins, 1989.

Morgan, GE, Mikhail MS: *Clinical Anesthesiology*, 1st ed., East Norwalk, CT, Appleton & Lange, 1992.

Morgan, GE, Mikhail MS: *Clinical Anesthesiology*, 2nd ed., East Norwalk, CT, Appleton & Lange, 1996.

Omoigui, S: *The Anesthesia Drug Handbook*, St. Louis, MO, Mosby-Year Book Inc., 1992.

Reed, AP: *Clinical Cases in Anesthesia*, 2nd ed., New York, Churchill Livingstone Inc., 1994.

Reed, AP, Kaplan JA: *Clinical Cases in Anesthesia*, New York, Churchill Livingstone Inc., 1989.

Rogers, MC et al.: *Principles and Practice of Anesthesiology*, St. Louis, MO, Mosby-Year Book Inc., 1993.

Stehling, L: *Common Problems in Pediatric Anesthesia*, 2nd ed., St. Louis, MO, Mosby-Year Book Inc., 1992.

Stoelting, RK, Dierdorf, SF: *Anethesia and Co-Existing Disease*, 3rd ed., New York, Churchill Livingstone Inc., 1993.

Stoelting, RK, Dierdorf, SF: *Handbook for Anesthesia and Co-Existing Disease*, New York, Churchill Livingstone Inc., 1993.

Stoelting, RK, Miller, RD: *Basics of Anesthesia*, 2nd ed. New York, Churchill Livingstone Inc., 1989.

Thaler, MS: *The Only EKG Book You'll Ever Need,* Philadelphia, J. B. Lippincott Company, 1988.

Yao, FF, Artusio, JF: *Anesthesiology: Problem-Oriented Patient Management*, 3rd ed., Philadelphia, J. B. Lippincott Company, 1993.